<u>Diabetes</u>
Overcome Your Fears

"So do not fear, for I am with you; do not be dismayed, for I am your God. I will strengthen you and help you; I will uphold you with my righteous right hand."

--Isaiah 41:10, NIV Bible

Diabetes

Overcome Your Fears

by D.R. Londrigan

Author's Note
This book is not intended as a substitute for professional medical care. The reader should work closely with a physician for all routine care and changes to their diabetes management program.

The author is grateful for permission to include the previously copyrighted material:
1. American Diabetes Association. "All About Diabetes." 2009. www.diabetes.org/about-diabetes.jsp. 16 June 2009.
2. American Diabetes Association. "The Dangerous Toll of Diabetes." 2009. www.diabetes.org/diabetes-statistics/dangerous-toll.jsp. 16 June 2009.
3. American Diabetes Association. "Diabetes Myths." 2009. www.diabetes.org/diabetes-myths.jsp. 16 June 2009. Copyright © 2009 American Diabetes Association.
From www.diabetes.org Reprinted with permission from *The American Diabetes Association.*

ISBN 978-0-615-32614-6

Published by DRL Publishing

Printed in the United States of America

Table of Contents

Introduction

Over the years, many people have encouraged me to write a book explaining my techniques for controlling my diabetes. Only in the last few years have I become aware of the tremendous need for such a book. I frequently encounter a fellow diabetic who is suffering needlessly, primarily because of confusion and a lack of education. Prior to deciding to write, I researched other resources available in order to determine the need. I was shocked to find that, even in this modern time, there are only a limited number of resources available that provide helpful information for controlling diabetes. Furthermore, many of these resources are overflowing with discouraging information. In fact, I found very few stories about long-time diabetics living a successful, healthy life. Toward the end of my search, I came across two particularly troubling issues. The first was a research article that claimed all diabetics had complications after 20 years of having the disease. I remember wondering that if I, a diabetic of 25 years, had no complications, as well as two others I know of, who have been diabetic for over 50 years each, hadn't been included in the statistics, how many others like us were out there to provide hope to others? Secondly, I encountered a man who was a Type 2 diabetic on pills. His doctor had not given him any idea how to improve his condition. He was left to try to develop a plan of care on his own. He had no idea that there was a chance that he could control his diabetes, prevent complications, and even eliminate his symptoms with some simple lifestyle changes.

I must preface by emphasizing that I am not a doctor, and am not, in any way medically trained. I am simply a long-time diabetic, with a great deal of life-experience. I have worked with many doctors, have personally dealt with the trial-and-error situations that a diabetic must contend with on a daily basis, and I have learned a few techniques to make these situations easier. This book is a compilation of advice and information that I have been given by doctors over the years, as well as my own personal research and experiences in living with the disease. I urge you to consult with your physician before making any changes based on the information you find in this book.

I have been so disheartened and frustrated over the years at the lack of encouraging information available. I think of diabetes like a game. According to Merriam-Webster's Dictionary, a game is defined in part as, "a procedure or strategy for gaining an end; … a physical or mental competition conducted according to rules with the participants in direct opposition to each other; …any activity undertaken or regarded as a contest involving rivalry, strategy, or struggle; area of expertise." Each of these definitions describes what diabetics must endure on a daily basis. The only way to maintain control is to continually develop strategies to overcome an opposing force, be it highs, lows, or diabetes in general. It is, no doubt, a struggle sometimes, and requires hard work and some expertise to "win" and survive the game. Taking control is possible though, if you know the "rules" of the game. The purpose of this book is to summarize those rules and details and clear up some confusing information you may have received, so you can live a healthier, more comfortable life. Because there are other resources available that will provide you with medical details and more scientific knowledge, this book is designed to provide the average person with a simple and basic understanding of diabetes and the strategies that can help prevent the disease from consuming your life. By taking charge of your body, you can have hope for a long and bright future.

1

"You have diabetes."

Because you are reading this book, chances are you have just heard those words. Whether the diagnosis has been given to you, your child, a close friend, or relative, you are likely concerned, scared to death, and unsure what to think. How serious is this disease? Is it curable? Are your children at risk? If you don't have children, will you be able to? Are complications a guarantee? What is the best way to get started caring for yourself (or someone close to you)? Outside of the medical jargon, just what do those words mean for you as a person? Just what is this monster named "diabetes" that has invaded your life without warning? The purpose of this book is to help answer those questions and give you hope in what may seem a bleak outlook.

My Story

My family was an average family. My father was in the Air Force, and my mom was a career woman, turned stay at home mom. My parents had me in their early twenties, and two and a half years later, my brother was born. Both are Christians, and they strived to raise us accordingly. We attended church regularly, with my parents working in the church throughout those years. It seemed life was going smoothly when we were all faced with one of the biggest hurdles of our lives.

I had been potty trained early on, but around my fourth birthday, I had begun bed-wetting and using the restroom with increasing frequency. Two weeks after I turned four, two incidences really got my parents' attention.

4

First, I took a very short nap one afternoon, during which I wet the bed. Then, I accompanied my mom on a shopping trip to the local mall. I was excessively thirsty, and I had to stop at every other store to use the restroom. She made an appointment and took me in, assuming I had a urinary tract infection that could be easily cured with antibiotics. The doctor ran a urine test and called my parents in for the results.

Dad had to work that day, and mom, confident it was nothing too serious, took me to my appointment. My mother has always thanked the Lord for the doctor she had that day, and she will never forget his kind words. "If this were 1926, I would have to tell you that your daughter has only six months to live. But, it is 1984, and there is no reason to think she won't live to be a happy, healthy grandmother. She has juvenile diabetes." Despite his kindness, she was left in total shock. As was standard at the time, I was admitted to the hospital for two weeks of tests and monitoring. Every four hours, a lab tech would come draw a tube of blood to run a blood glucose (BG) test. Finally, they inserted a heparin lock (similar to an I.V. catheter) into my wrist, which was then used to allow blood draws for the tests. I was put on insulin injections. I was finally released from the hospital on a prescribed regimen of four BG tests per day and one insulin injection every morning.

The only diabetic we knew at the time was my paternal grandfather, who was a very unhealthy, Type 2 diabetic. As a result of his obesity and inactive lifestyle, his diabetes had resulted in several complications over the years. He was legally blind, suffered from heart disease, arteriosclerosis, and neuropathy. My parents did not want me to wind up in his condition, so they demanded the most modern and accurate equipment available at the time. In 1984, there was a limited selection of equipment options. I tested with one of the first styles of home meters produced, and it cost around $250. The strip was about four inches long, had two color-change pads on top, and required a very large drop of blood. The test took two minutes and gave a digital read-out. Thus began our journey into the world of diabetes.

Within a few months of my diagnosis, my father was deployed to Korea for a year. This left my mother home to care for a newly-diagnosed four-year-old and my two-year-old brother. Not sure how to handle the stress of being a single parent with no family nearby to turn to for help, she consulted my doctor. He suggested that she teach me how to care for myself. She did. At four years of age, I learned how to test my blood sugar, draw up my insulin into the syringe, and give my own shot. Of course, mom was looking over my shoulder the whole time. I have always been thankful for her choice. Because she was willing to hand over that responsibility, I felt like I was in control of my disease, rather then my disease being in control of me. My parents also taught me a phrase that the doctor had said to them during the initial diagnosis. "You are not a diabetic; rather you happen to have diabetes."

Mom did everything possible to arrange for me to be as "normal" as possible. If I stayed with someone for any extended period, she would teach them to give injections by having them practice injecting an orange first, then actually sticking her arm. Each year before the school term began, she held a meeting with the school nurses, principal, and teachers to educate them and discuss an emergency plan. She would teach me responses to questions by other kids who were concerned about "catching" my diabetes, such as, "Well, diabetes is like a broken leg. Something in my body is broken, but you can't catch it." One year, when I had a teacher who rewarded students with candy, Mom gave her a supply of sugarless candy for me. Mom generally prepared my lunches, but for the occasional school lunch I purchased, she educated me on dietary needs. I could only have specific amounts of carbs, but all the protein and vegetables I wanted. I was only allowed skim milk. If we had cake at a party, I had to scrape the icing off. When donuts were served, I had to eat the plain cake donut with no topping or topped with just peanuts. I was allowed two slices of pizza, and no dessert, or one slice and a little dessert. I could have a small portion of plain ice cream, but no sugary toppings. I was occasionally allowed sweets to treat a low blood sugar, but otherwise, my diet was relatively strict. Both my parents held me accountable for eating the wrong thing. In our house, "snitching" sweets was a major sin! They taught me early on that I would be the one who would eventually suffer the consequences. However, and I consider this a very important point, after they taught me, they trusted me to make my own decisions. They did an amazing job of not making me feel trapped, over-protected, or "different." They also taught me that diabetes was a minor inconvenience compared to what some people experience.

For several years, I attended a summer camp for permanently disabled children. By the end of camp each year, I had new friends suffering from conditions such as cerebral palsy, epilepsy, lung and heart conditions, physical disfigurements, mental conditions, or combinations of the above. I realized at a young age that I was a very blessed person, and had no right to feel sorry for myself. I also attended several children's diabetes camps, where I learned that, with preparation, I could do whatever I set my mind to do. Of course, I still had my ups and downs.

My parents worked closely with my doctors, and they strived hard to help me maintain good BGs and Hemoglobin A1Cs (a test that shows an average measurement of your blood glucose levels for the previous six weeks. A "normal" result is typically a number between 5.0 and 6.0, while a diabetic's results are generally recommended to be between 6.0 and 7.0). Despite their diligent efforts, my blood sugars were often a roller coaster. I was eventually put on a regimen of two shots each day, one in the morning, and one in the evening. While on vacation one summer, I was so excited to leave camp that morning to go to an amusement park, I forgot to take my morning shot. After drinking two 32-ounce drinks in a row, followed by a vomiting spell afterward, we realized my unquenchable thirst was a direct result of the forgotten shot. I was in ketoacidosis (a condition caused by a shortage of available glucose, in which the body breaks down proteins and fats). In addition, over the years I had several severe lows, two resulting in trips to the emergency room for intravenous dextrose (which raises blood sugar rapidly). I will always remember one particular event, in which the excitement of the day caused multiple low BGs that would not come up, despite our efforts. Unfortunately, we were on an airplane at the time, and my sugar continued to drop lower. By the time we landed, I was low enough that an ambulance was called to unload me from the plane and rush me to the hospital for monitoring. I was fully conscious the entire time, so you can imagine the embarrassment I felt in being so helpless in the situation.

Illness was another issue I learned to deal with. Unlike most kids, I loved to get sick! When I would catch some type of stomach bug, it meant I could have a sugary "sick-day diet," as prescribed by my doctor. I could have things normally forbidden, such as Lifesavers' candies, Jell-O, Gatorade, Sprite, and 7-up. It was the only way to keep my sugar up since I still had to take my shots, and I am sure I feigned an inability to eat normal foods a time or two because of it. One day, however, I couldn't even stomach the sweet sodas. I quickly became dehydrated and risked a severe low. Mom and Dad took me to the hospital, where a young doctor mistakenly gave me an I.V. drip of dextrose solution rather than saline (my BG was not actually low at the time, therefore a saline solution should have been administered rather than the high-sugar dextrose). A few minutes later, a lab tech drew a blood sample, and the results showed my BG skyrocketed to 1200—about 12 times the normal level. How I was still conscious nobody knows, but we assume the result had to have been inaccurate due to the fact the blood was drawn from the same arm and directly upstream from the I.V. drip.

By the time I was in third grade, I had become more conscious of my limitations and differences, and I decided I wanted to be as normal as possible. So I quit testing my blood sugars. I don't recall how long this rebellion lasted; I think it was a matter of days. Interestingly, I continued my insulin regimen, but as far as testing, I became an instantaneous master at deceiving my parents into thinking I was perfectly fine. Mom would periodically remind me to test, and I would arrange to disappear to my bedroom for about two minutes (the length of time my meter took to give a result). I would then walk out and tell her a number I knew sounded realistic. One evening, she told me to go test. I made the mistake of coming out of my room too soon. I gave her a number in the 120's. She was instantly suspicious and asked me to bring her the strip I had just used. I went and dug frantically through my trash can in search of a strip with pads the color of the 120's range. I finally chose one, but mom immediately saw that it lacked the fresh sheen of a recently used strip, and asked how long I had been lying. That was the end of my rebellion, but not my punishment. For quite some time after that, I had to test with supervision, and, even worse, I had to confess to my doctors. I don't remember what they said to me, but I vaguely remember a short, but kind lecture from one doctor explaining the results of not caring for myself. Perhaps she also explained the alternative if I did take care of myself. In any case, I decided then that I would do better.

I learned another important lesson when I was in fifth grade. My class recessed with the fourth graders, and the fourth grade teacher had been my favorite. I loved her, and I knew the feeling was mutual. When April Fool's day arrived, my fifth grade teacher tried to convince me to act like my sugar was low, and when he signaled me, to pretend to pass out. It was to be his joke of the year towards her. I tried to explain that my parents had told me to never pretend such things, but he eventually convinced me to do it. I will never forget the look of panic and terror in that poor woman's eyes, or the fear I saw in the eyes of my classmates who quickly gathered around. I never pretended such things again.

When I hit my teen years, I got a new BG meter that only took 45 seconds. At this time, the insulin pump was new technology. My parents did their research, decided they wanted me on it, and talked to doctors. Insurance, however, refused to pay for it unless it was "medically necessary." The insurance company required a documented, physical reason I couldn't use injections. Interestingly, within a few months, my annual urine test resulted in the discovery that I had microscopic kidney damage. My doctor and parents used that diagnosis to convince the insurance company to cover the pump. They were successful, and I got my first pump when I was 15. Because the technology was still relatively new, and my doctor was still learning about it herself, I was admitted to the hospital for a 72 hour monitoring. I wasn't allowed to administer any boluses or corrections without medical supervision, and had to test every two hours. A diabetes educator taught me how to read food labels, count carbohydrates, and estimate meal carbs. I went home on the pump, absolutely thrilled with my new-found freedom. In order to celebrate, my dad decided to take me out for a real treat. He took me to the local ice cream shop for a Sundae. When we arrived, he asked me what kind I wanted. We both realized then that I didn't know what a Sundae was, and therefore, had no idea what I wanted on it. That is when it hit us both how wonderful the pump truly was. That's not to say the pump allowed total freedom to eat what I pleased, rather, we realized the possibilities and experiences that were potentially available with it. Over the next year, I was able to stabilize my BG levels and lower my Hemoglobin A1C. As a direct result of the increased control, the following year's urine test showed that my kidneys had healed, and there was no longer any sign of damage.

Teenage hormones are tricky under normal conditions, but when a permanent medical condition is added to the mix, they can make life downright miserable. Like all teenage girls, I became interested in boys. But when year after year went by with hardly a glance, let alone a date, I started to feel very self-conscious. A few times, I tried asking boys out, and typically got turned down. I felt my disease was scaring boys away. I began trying to hide in bathrooms to test my sugar or even take a bolus with my pump. My high school's lunch program made things even worse. Because of the limited time they allowed for lunch, I often didn't get to eat my full lunch. To solve that problem and prevent low sugars later, I had to leave my class five minutes early to get to the lunch room before the other kids. This fact added a lot of jealousy and unwanted attention to the mix. I suspect my self-esteem was low enough by that point, it affected the way everyone saw me. I was convinced no guy could see past my condition to love me enough to be interested in dating or marrying me. I had also grown up in an era that believed diabetic women *do not* have babies. So as a blossoming teenager, there I was, feeling like I didn't have a friend in the world, convinced I would never get married or have kids. Everywhere I turned, it seemed like I heard how complications were inevitable with diabetes. The seemingly imminent complications scared me, and there were many nights I laid in bed and cried, wishing I could just die.

Fortunately, I stayed involved in church. Through my youth group and youth conferences I attended, I realized that God had a plan for me, despite how useless I felt. I convinced myself there was a reason He had allowed me to have this disease. I realized that, if I would let Him, God could potentially use my disease for something great one day. I made the decision then to accept my disease and see where God led. I resolved to turn my attention away from boys for the most part, and focus on a passion I had had for years—animals.

I began volunteering at local horse barns and veterinary clinics. Eventually, I got my own horses, and began training horses for others. I worked as a veterinary technician, and even became a puppy-raiser for a guide dog program. I was still somewhat convinced that, based on statistics, I would go blind within a few more years. So, deep inside, I thought that by raising and training the puppies, maybe I could get my foot in the door to have a seeing-eye dog in the future. I went to college and majored in Animal Biology and Pre-veterinary Sciences. Although I still dreamed of getting married one day, I had resolved myself to go to vet school and be content as a single career woman. My life was mapped out, and I was on my way. Or so I thought.

I was 20 years old when I moved out of my parents' house. We were all nervous, of course. Because of my incredible sensitivity to activity, stress, and emotions, I was considered a "brittle" diabetic. I could get low very easily and very quickly. They made me promise to always test my blood sugar before driving. Shortly before moving out, I had two particularly severe lows during the night. My mom and brother found me the next morning when I didn't awake to go to school. Thank the Lord, they were able to wake me, but I was extremely combative and they had to force me to drink some juice. Due to these episodes in particular, we agreed that I would call home first thing every morning so they could make sure I had awakened that morning. A severe nighttime low was always a threat and those calls were a cruel reminder of my mortality that I tried not to think about in my desire for independence. At the same time, however, I found comfort in the fact that if I missed a call, my parents would arrange for help within a short time-frame. After moving out, I became very active in my church's singles' group, and spent several evenings a week participating in the singles' activities. I went on a few dates with guys from the group, but remained focused on my schooling and career. I was content to just have friends.

One guy in that group quickly became my best friend. We were always together, but never more than friends. He was comfortable with my diabetes, and we had a great deal in common. He was also in the Air Force, and familiar with the lifestyle in which I had grown up. Eventually, we started dating. When I realized our relationship was getting more serious, I confided to him one evening that I would not be able to have children. Knowing that he dreamed of several, I dreaded his response. He lovingly put his arm around me and said, "OK, if we decide we want children, we can always look into adoption." Within a year of meeting, we were engaged. Suddenly, my path totally changed, and I realized that it was possible for someone other than my parents to see past my disability.

We married, and our honeymoon included some high-energy activities, such as cave spelunking, rock climbing, white-water rafting, hiking, and other activities. My new husband was eager to learn about my diabetes and how to care for me in an emergency. He was always packing extra juice for the strenuous activities, and double-checking to make sure I had all my testing supplies. He was understanding and patient when I had a low, and was always quick to help me if I needed assistance.

As a part of our new-found marriage relationship, we were faced with how to deal with diabetes and intimacy. There were many nights where, just after setting the "mood", the activities of the day would affect me, and my blood sugar would drop quickly. Some nights I recovered quickly enough to continue enjoying the moment, but other times would take much longer, and he would fall asleep before I got my sugar stabilized. Those nights were humiliating. The pump itself was an issue I was very self-conscious about. Some nights I was able to plan for an intimate time, in which case, I would remove the whole set. Spontaneous moments, however, resulted in us having to figure out whether or not my sugar was stable enough to disconnect, and if not, where to lay the pump so it was out of our way. Though it took a while for me to adjust to the embarrassment of such moments, it helped tremendously that my husband was so understanding. If he sensed I was self-conscious or embarrassed, he was quick to remind me that he loved me the way I was, pump and all. As far as he was concerned, the pump and my disease were a part of me, and he loved me despite inconvenient tubes, low blood sugars, and poorly timed BG tests.

I was very fortunate to marry a health-nut. My husband is very active, and eats very healthy, well-balanced, and nutritious meals. Although I was raised somewhat strictly, I was never as healthy as he encouraged me to be. It took some time for me to adjust to eating his diet, but I knew it was best for me. I continued working with horses, which kept me active. I also became a puppy-raiser again for Guide Dogs for the Blind. My doctor had helped get my BGs under tight control, and, after living this improved lifestyle for several months, my Hemoglobin A1C test showed a drop to 6.5. When I approached the idea of having children, my doctor was very supportive. She explained that, as long as I kept my blood sugars under control, ate healthy, worked closely with specialists, and had no complications to begin with, there was no reason I couldn't have perfectly healthy pregnancies and babies. I relayed this information to my husband, and he was thrilled. So we decided to go for it, but we wanted to plan it carefully.

My doctor recommended a full physical and lab panel for me, to make sure there were no complications. To my surprise, the urine test results showed that I was in stage one renal failure. I did not want to risk worsening the damage by getting pregnant, so I put pregnancy on the back-burner for a while. I knew that I had reversed kidney damage years before, and although the first time was less serious, I thought it was worth a try. For the next four months I really tightened my control on my blood sugars. I decided I didn't want my BG, HgbA1C, cholesterols, and other related tests to be the often recommended "target levels for diabetics." Rather, I wanted to target the levels of normal, healthy people. It wasn't easy, and I had some ups and downs, but by the end of the four-month period, my HgbA1C was 5.8, my BGs were consistently between 85 and 120, and I felt wonderful. When the urine test was run again about eight months later, the results came back clean, showing no signs of damage.

So, we again discussed the possibility of pregnancy with my doctor, who fully supported us. She recommended a perinatologist who was experienced in pregnant women with Type 1 diabetes, and we began our journey to parenthood. Within a few months, I was pregnant. Like most new parents-to-be, we were elated and scared to death at the same time. However, we had the additional fears of diabetes-related complications. We lived almost two hours from my doctor and the hospital where I was scheduled to deliver. Because my doctors wanted to monitor me and the pregnancy closely, I had to make the trip twice a month until I was 20 weeks gestation, and every week thereafter. This took a great deal of dedication, but every visit allowed me a chance to see a brief ultrasound of the baby I was carrying. A baby that I thought I would never have; yet, there it was, kicking mightily.

Early in the pregnancy, it occurred to me that, until that time, no one had been dependent on me. My husband was frequently away on military assignments, leaving me home alone for days or weeks at a time. Should a situation arise where I passed out or just didn't wake up one morning, no other lives were at risk. Yet, in a matter of a few months, there would be a baby whose life would be affected, and that scared me to death!

Because of the Guide Dog program we were involved in, I was heavily involved in Service Dog education at the time. While researching a project one day, I found some information about Medical Alert Dogs for Diabetes. These dogs were specifically trained to alert the diabetic owner to a low blood sugar, before the person was at risk of the BG level dropping too low. I was fascinated and excited at the possibility. After a great deal of research into the legal aspects, I found an experienced trainer for alert dogs, and, with her help, purchased and began training my first alert dog, a Golden Retriever named Jack. Soon, my new dog was alerting to low blood sugars on a regular basis.

My early pregnancy was, for the most part, uneventful. I had some severe round ligament pains early on, but by limiting my activities somewhat, the pain diminished. As the pregnancy progressed, I was continually educating myself, and doing what I could to keep tight control of my sugar levels. The 16 week triple screen test showed everything was fine, and by the end of the second trimester, my HgbA1C was 5.6. Around 28 weeks gestation, the baby suddenly started growing quickly, despite my well-controlled blood sugars. At 32 weeks, I started having contractions, was rushed to the hospital, and treatments began for pre-term labor. I was put on a magnesium I.V. drip for several days, and hospitalized, on bed rest, for the following week. Once the contractions were stabilized, I was sent home on a muscle relaxer and strict orders for a modified bed rest. Shortly after arriving back home, I developed an intense itch that rapidly spread over most of my body. When a rash began forming in my stretch marks, the doctor diagnosed me with Pruritic Urticarial Papules and Plaques of Pregnancy (PUPPP), an uncommon and torturous, pregnancy-induced rash. My doctor explained that the only cure was to have the baby. So for the next few weeks, I just had to wait it out and try not to scratch too much. As if that wasn't enough, I noticed at 33 weeks that my body was becoming increasingly resistant to insulin. My daily requirement tripled, and I had frequent highs after eating. My doctor put me on a high-protein and vegetable diet, with just enough carbohydrates to keep baby and myself healthy. By 36 weeks, the physical stress of the pregnancy combined with the emotional stress of the insulin resistance, PUPPP rash and itch, and bed rest finally took its toll and sent me into pre-term labor once again. We drove to the hospital, where I was admitted for monitoring.

After arriving at the hospital, the contractions eased somewhat, but the doctor was concerned about the continuous contractions (several contractions per hour for four weeks at this point) beginning to stress the baby. He decided to perform an amniocentesis to check the baby's lung development. The results showed that it was safe to deliver the baby. The final ultrasound, however, showed the baby was quite large in comparison to my pelvis. Because I was only 36 weeks along, however, we agreed to try for an induced vaginal birth. After laboring for some time, the baby's head lodged in my pelvis. I was rushed to the operating room for an emergency cesarean section. Finally, after everything I'd gone through, we had a beautiful, perfectly healthy little boy. Interestingly enough, there was no indication that my complications were related to being diabetic. Rather, the pre-term labor and difficult delivery issues seemed to be a result of a genetically large baby, and my body just couldn't handle that size well. The doctor felt I had a great chance of normal future pregnancies.

About eight months later, through some unexpected circumstances, we acquired a dog named Will, who began learning how to alert from Jack. When he showed promising signs of becoming a service animal, I felt I needed to arrange to place one of the dogs with another diabetic. We decided to make arrangements for Jack to go, as he was alerting consistently. I would then encourage and improve Will's training as a Medical Alert and Response Service Dog. Within a year, Will was alerting, retrieving juice boxes when I had a low sugar, and assisting me in several other ways. I began researching Alert Dog schools in order to get him certified. In the mean time, I continued to focus on my family and controlling my diabetes while raising a child.

I learned so much about my body while pregnant with my son, that keeping my sugars under tight control afterwards was much easier. By the time he was a year old, my HgbA1C's were consistently between 5.2 and 5.6. We decided to pursue a second baby. I talked to my doctors, had a full physical and lab panel run to check for any unknown complications, and we were given the go ahead. Shortly thereafter, I was pregnant, but miscarried within a few weeks. Again, it was deemed unrelated to my diabetes. We waited the suggested time, and I was soon pregnant with our second child.

Like my first pregnancy, I had to make frequent trips to my doctors and had severe round ligament pain. This time around, however, I was more relaxed since I knew what was happening. Also, like the first pregnancy, we took the screening test at 16 weeks gestation, in order to test for any potential complications. This time, though, the results showed that I had an increased risk for pregnancy complications. The doctor told me to continue doing things as I had been, and just be aware of any changes. Things continued uneventfully until I reached 23 weeks, when I suddenly experienced a few hard contractions. I called the doctor, and he prescribed the same muscle relaxers from my first pregnancy. At 26 weeks, my blood pressure increased slightly, so I was ordered to go on a modified bed rest. At 28 weeks, the contractions became more regular, so the bed rest became more strict. Over the next few weeks, I again experienced the increasing insulin resistance and had to return to the high-protein, low-carb diet. Then, at 34 weeks, I noticed a decrease in resistance. I casually mentioned it to my doctor at the 35 week appointment, and he became concerned. Apparently the decrease in insulin resistance was a strong indication of premature placental deterioration. He gave me instructions to watch for some symptoms such as further decreasing BG levels. Within 48 hours, I had experienced the symptoms and was immediately hospitalized and put on fetal monitors. The monitor showed the baby was still OK, so the doctor ran an amniocentesis to check the lung development.

According to the results, the lungs were not developed enough for an ideal birth, and delivering the baby meant the possibility of a long-term stay in the Neonatal Intensive Care Unit (NICU). The doctor decided to keep me hooked to the fetal monitors, on strict bed rest, and try to wait a bit longer before delivering. God provided, and my body held out. The day I hit 37 weeks, I was taken into the operating room and the baby delivered. We were blessed with a gorgeous, healthy, baby girl. Once again, there was no real explanation for the pre-term contractions. The placental issue is a known risk of diabetic pregnancies, but everything was fine after the baby was delivered.

Because of the difficulties of my pregnancies, my doctors recommended I not get pregnant again. We desired more children though, so we decided to adopt. In 2008, we adopted a beautiful, newborn baby boy. His birthmother had not received early pre-natal care, and after arriving at the hospital late in her third trimester, it was discovered that she had gestational diabetes and severe pre-eclampsia. The doctors decided to perform an emergency c-section to stabilize the mother's condition. When the baby was born, he showed the classic signs of a mother with uncontrolled diabetes. He was a large, fat baby, weighing almost 10 pounds. Furthermore, despite a dextrose I.V., his blood sugar levels would not rise above 50 for three days, and did not stabilize in a normal range for five days. Because of the low blood sugars, and several other minor complications, he was very weak for a few days and had trouble eating. Fortunately, after spending a week in the NICU, he improved and was able to come home with us. Nonetheless, it was very interesting being able to compare the results of well-controlled diabetes with uncontrolled diabetes.

As of this writing, I have been a Type 1 diabetic for 25 years, on the pump for about 15 years, and still have no complications. I have been married for over seven years, and I have given birth to two beautiful children, neither having developed diabetes at this writing. We have adopted two children, and are open to the idea of adopting again in the future. I currently strive to maintain my BGs between 80 and 110 and HgbA1Cs between 5.5 and 6.0. I have upgraded my medical equipment several times over the years, and am currently using the latest in insulin pump technology and a meter that takes only five seconds. I occasionally use a Continuous Glucose Monitoring System to re-stabilize my BG levels when necessary. I have retired my Medical Alert Service Dog from official duty, but he still chooses to alert to occasional low sugars at home. My family is active, and I stay busy with my four children.

2

What is diabetes?

I am assuming you have heard plenty of medical terminology and "official" medical descriptions of the disease by now. Based on my experience however, far too many newly-diagnosed diabetics and their loved ones still do not understand the disease and what exactly the diagnosis means. Furthermore, as a diabetic, you will often hear terms such as "Pre-diabetic," "Type 1," "Type 2," and "Gestational" to describe the type of diabetes one has.

According to the nation's leading diabetes research organization, the American Diabetes Association, "there are 20.8 million children and adults in the United States, or 7% of the population, who have diabetes. While an estimated 14.6 million have been diagnosed with diabetes, unfortunately, 6.2 million people (or nearly one-third) are unaware that they have the disease.... There are 54 million Americans who have pre-diabetes, in addition to the 20.8 million with diabetes."[1] Of these 20.8 million, about 90-95% of diabetics are Type 2 [2]. In this chapter, I will explain, in very simplistic terms, what diabetes is, as well as the different types. Note that there is a great deal more involved than will be discussed in this chapter, but this is designed to give you a simple understanding of the basics of diabetes.

There are basically two types of diabetes, Type 1, also known as Juvenile Diabetes, and Type 2, often known as Adult-Onset. A third variation, known as Gestational Diabetes, is considered a version of Type 2 that affects only pregnant women. In recent years, due to the fact that more children and teenagers are being diagnosed with Type 2, the term "Adult Onset" is almost unheard today. The confusing thing about Type 1 and Type 2 diabetes is, although they share a similar name and even similar symptoms, they have very different causes. A friend, who is a physician, explained the difference as, "Type 1 means no insulin is produced, while Type 2 means too much insulin is produced." This is a great way to picture it, however, there is much more involved. Before you can understand diabetes, you must understand how a "normal," healthy body works.

The body contains a multitude of systems that work together to keep you alive. Examples of these systems are the digestive system, which digests food to allow it to be absorbed into the blood stream; the respiratory system, which exchanges used air for new air in order to supply your cells with oxygen; the endocrine system, which is primarily responsible for hormone production; and the cardiovascular system, which keeps blood pumping throughout your body, and carries the air, water, nutrients, and other necessities to every cell. The cardiovascular system is literally the "highway system" that carries everything and sustains the body. Another important system is the nervous system, which is responsible for relaying "messages" of touch, smell, sight, taste, temperature, pain, and other signals between the brain and the individual parts of the body.

The endocrine system performs multiple functions. The pancreas is one organ of the endocrine system, and performs several important jobs. One job is completed by specialized cells in the pancreas known as islet cells, which produce insulin. There is normally a steady supply of glucose found in the bloodstream. The main purpose of insulin is to help cells of the body absorb sugars from the bloodstream by opening "pathways" through the cell membranes. To help keep the level balanced, the pancreas periodically releases minute amounts of insulin throughout the day. This amount is referred to as a "basal" rate, or the base amount required to maintain proper levels. There is a second type of release, known as a "bolus." A bolus of insulin is a larger amount that is released based on a sudden surge of glucose in the bloodstream. Almost everything that a person eats or drinks has some amount of sugar in it. Sugars come in different forms, and through the digestive process, they are transformed into a usable form called glucose. The glucose and other nutrients are then absorbed into the bloodstream. The insulin allows the glucose to be absorbed from the bloodstream into the cells.

In a healthy body, as glucose levels in the bloodstream rise, the pancreas releases insulin into the bloodstream to increase cell absorption and stabilize and maintain the glucose at a healthy level in the blood. If glucose levels begin to decline, insulin production slows temporarily to ensure the blood glucose levels are not exhausted. If the glucose cannot leave the bloodstream and levels get too high, it is considered a *hyper*glycemic condition, and, over time, can affect the body in many ways, ultimately causing complications such as retinopathy, heart disease, and much more. This is also known as "insulin resistance," because "pathways" between bloodstream and cells resist being opened without large amounts of insulin. On the other hand, if there is too much insulin for the amount of glucose available, the pathways become very sensitive and open easily, the blood glucose levels in the bloodstream may fall too low, and it is considered a *hypo*glycemic reaction. This starves the cells of essential nutrients, and as a result, the brain and other important organs cease to function properly. Within a very short amount of time, the organs can begin to shut down, eventually causing permanent brain damage and even death.

Other factors also affect glucose and insulin levels. Factors such as exercise, stress, weight, and hormones affect how quickly cells absorb glucose and how much insulin is required. In addition to the pancreas, the liver also assists in stabilizing insulin levels. One of the liver's functions is to store a certain amount of glucose in the form of glycogen. Any excess sugar consumed is stored either in the liver or in fat cells. In the event the blood glucose level drops too low, the liver will convert the excess glycogen into glucose and release it into the bloodstream. Based on the amount released, the pancreas will then counteract the excess glucose with insulin.

Blood glucose, or BG, levels are typically measured in milligrams of glucose per deciliter of blood, or mg/dl. A normal healthy body generally maintains a BG level of 80 – 100 mg/dl. When the body has a frequent BG level above or below this normal level, the person is typically diagnosed as hypoglycemic, hyperglycemic, or diabetic. Testing for diabetes is relatively simple. One commonly used test is the Oral Glucose Tolerance Test, in which "a person's blood glucose level is measured after a fast and two hours after drinking a glucose-rich beverage. If the two-hour blood glucose level is between 140 and 199 mg/dl, the person tested has pre-diabetes. If the two-hour blood glucose level is at 200 mg/dl or higher, the person tested has diabetes." [1]. As a side note, there is currently a push by some medical professionals to begin using the Hemoglobin A1C test as a more accurate diabetes diagnostic tool, as the HA1C gives a better analysis of BG levels over a longer period of time.

Because the majority of diabetics (about 90-95%) have Type 2, I will explain it first. There are certainly exceptions in which people become resistant to insulin due to other issues, however, most of the time Type 2 is caused by a person's lifestyle choices. While genetics can pre-dispose a person to the potential of developing the disease, it is usually very preventable. Generally speaking, a Type 2 diabetic is a person who eats a high-carbohydrate diet and has a low activity level. As a result, they tend to gain weight. Remember that exercise, hormones, weight, and stress are a few factors that affect insulin production and absorption. So when a person eats a high-carb diet, high levels of insulin must be produced to counteract the resulting glucose. As the high-carb diet continues, the person will generally gain weight. As weight increases, additional fat cells are produced. As additional cells are produced, more insulin is needed to open the added "pathways", and the pathways themselves become more resistant to the insulin. The additional weight also makes activity uncomfortable, so the activity level typically decreases. As activity decreases, weight increases. As weight continues to increase, hormone levels are affected, which causes physical and emotional stress. As more insulin is needed, and as it becomes harder for the glucose to be absorbed from the bloodstream, insulin resistance increases. This snowball affect continues until the pancreas can no longer produce the amount of insulin required. At that point, BG levels begin to rise, and the person may be diagnosed as "pre-diabetic." If nothing is done to decrease blood sugars and they continue to rise, then the insulin-producing cells of the pancreas will become very overworked, and damage will begin to occur. The person will be diagnosed as a "Type 2 diabetic."

A person with Type 2 diabetes often experiences symptoms such as increased thirst, irritable moods, headaches, vision changes, and an increased need to urinate. Most doctors prescribe a change in lifestyle first, including recommending a lower-carb diet, weight loss, and exercise. While there may always be an increased risk of re-developing Type 2 diabetes, in many cases, the symptoms of Type 2 diabetes can be totally eliminated if the person can change their lifestyle and improve their health. If the person chooses to continue an unhealthy lifestyle, or, for some other reason is considered incurable with lifestyle changes alone, then the doctor will prescribe some form of medication. The purpose of the medication is to help the body absorb the available insulin, thereby decreasing resistance. If that doesn't work, then a regimen of daily insulin injections will be prescribed in order to make up for the increased need. It is possible, that, over time, the pancreas will literally wear out, and insulin production will stop altogether. If this occurs, daily insulin via injections or the pump is required. Although the disease becomes almost identical to Type 1 at this stage (and some doctors even refer to it as Type 1), technically, it is still Type 2 diabetes due to the original cause.

Gestational diabetics are similar to Type 2 diabetics because the condition is caused by insulin resistance. The condition is generally diagnosed in the third trimester of pregnancy. This is when pregnancy hormones increase, and in many cases, carb intake and weight also increase, while activity level decreases. In addition, the growing placenta absorbs a large amount of the insulin produced. As a result, insulin resistance increases. Due to the pregnancy, diet and exercise cannot typically be recommended, and most medications are not considered safe during pregnancy. Therefore, the patient is usually prescribed insulin injections from the beginning. Once the baby is born, the placenta is no longer a factor, and diet, activity level, and hormones often return to normal. In most cases, the woman will return to her normal, healthy, non-diabetic state soon after birth. On occasion, however, the resistance will continue. This is usually due to an unhealthy amount of weight gain during the pregnancy. At this point, the woman may be diagnosed as having Type 2.

Type 1 is quite a different story. It is more commonly diagnosed in children and teens under the age of 18, though, on occasion, adults of all ages may develop it as well. The ultimate cause of Type 1 is still unknown. A great deal of research and studies are ongoing in the hope of finding the cause; however, there are several theories that support potential causes. To summarize the explanations my doctors have provided me over the years, genetics seem to play a part, in that the person has received a genetically faulty immune system. Most doctors agree that Type 1 is an immune disorder, and many hold the belief that a severe illness will trigger the immune system. Occasionally, for some unknown reason, the immune response then turns on itself and begins to destroy necessary body cells. For example, a child may develop chicken pox, measles, or some other severe viral or bacterial infection, and the immune system begins fighting the infection. Whatever the reason for the immune response, for some unknown reason, the body then turns on itself and begins to kill islet cells. For a period of time, often called the "honeymoon period," the pancreas still has some functioning islet cells producing insulin. Within a short time, however – typically a few months—the immune system kills all the islet cells. Currently, we cannot safely alter the immune responses, so there is no way to stop this attack on the islet cells. As the cells are destroyed, insulin supplies in the bloodstream rapidly decrease, and BG levels increase. Like other types of diabetics, the patient will often begin to notice increased thirst, urination, vision changes, moodiness, and headaches. In some cases, particularly with children, BG levels consistently over 120 often result in a diagnosis of Type 1. On occasion, levels may climb so quickly, the child suffers a seizure or other problem before the parents realize there is a problem. It is common for children to arrive at the emergency room with BG levels well over 300. A Type 1 patient is immediately prescribed insulin injections and BG monitoring. At this time, there is no approved cure for Type 1 diabetes.

Nothing a person does or does not do will affect whether or not they develop the disease. While there are tests that can rate the predisposition of a child to develop diabetes, there is no test that will give a definitive answer as to whether or when the child will develop the disease. As an additional note, the term "brittle diabetic" is frequently used, and often misunderstood. The best explanation I ever heard for this term came from a doctor-friend who said that brittleness is based on your degree of sensitivity to things. With Type 1, either you are in control or you are not. Brittleness has nothing to do with control; rather, it refers to how your body reacts to other factors. For example, I strive for very tight control, with my BG levels between 80 and 120 the majority of the time. However, I am highly sensitive to factors such as hormones, activity, and acute stress—factors which may be out of my control. For example, when I exercise, although I turn my insulin off entirely for more strenuous activities, I may still experience a low. I am also very sensitive to insulin itself. It takes very little insulin to drop my BG levels quite significantly. Obviously, this sensitivity can result in dramatically fluctuating BG levels, but it is the sensitivity causing the fluctuating BG levels that is considered "brittle," rather than the BG levels themselves.

Newly diagnosed patients generally experience similar symptoms, despite the type of diabetes they have. However, the longer the person has the disease, the more variable, and personal, the symptoms become. Symptoms of a high blood sugar may involve one or more symptoms, to include headaches, increased thirst and urination, persistent fungal or bacterial infections, vision changes, moodiness, forgetfulness, an overall "blah" feeling, bad taste in the mouth, sweet-smelling breath, and, eventually, ketoacidosis, seizures, coma, and death. The treatment for high BG levels is to administer insulin to allow the absorption of excess glucose from the bloodstream into the cells. On the other hand, common symptoms of a low blood sugar include adrenalin-type responses such as sweating and shakiness, an inability to focus, decreased cognitive ability, overall weakness and lack of energy, moodiness, vision changes, hunger, and eventually seizure, coma, and death. "The better your glucose control, the less likely you are to develop complications of diabetes." [3]

3

So Now What?

There are numerous scientific and medical diabetes books available, and I encourage you to do some research. The best way to take control of your diabetes, rather than have it control you, is to be informed. Because of other resources available, I am going to limit this chapter to tips, suggestions, and observations based on my personal experiences and research, and questions I have frequently heard from other diabetics. I have found them helpful over the years, and I hope they will help you as well.

Your first step as a newly diagnosed diabetic is to find a good doctor. Because I grew up in the military, and married military, I have moved and had to change doctors many times throughout my life. I have learned a few things over the years that may prevent you from becoming the next "experiment" for your doctor. I have had doctors who, on my first visit, would instruct me to make changes to my insulin that resulted in my almost perfectly controlled blood sugars going absolutely haywire. Alternately, I have had doctors who, after one visit, could transform my roller-coaster BGs into perfectly controlled levels, with just a few tweaks to my insulin rates. I have had one doctor who would forget to even look at my BG records during my appointment, another who admitted after several months that he didn't know how to help me gain the tight control I wanted, and yet another who sent me out of his office in tears because he was so adamantly opposed to the tight control I had. That may sound strange, but I have encountered several doctors like this one over the years who prefer their patients keep their BGs relatively high (150-200 mg/dl range) in order to give them a wide "buffer" to prevent lows. Yet another doctor, and his staff, actually pretended to be diabetic for a week or so at a time, taking saline injections and/or wearing a saline pump and testing their BGs regularly. This allowed them to be more understanding and empathetic toward their patients. So, with the wide selection of doctor personalities and preferences out there, how do you find one that has your best interest in mind?

Start by deciding what your personal goals are. Through various studies, the American Diabetes Association has determined that, "The closer your A1C is to the normal range (less than six percent), the lower your chances of complications. However, you increase your risk of hypoglycemia, especially if you have Type 1 diabetes"[3]. Do you want to aim for "normal" BG levels and Hemoglobin A1C's at the risk of frequent, potentially severe lows, or would you prefer elevated BGs and HgbA1C's to prevent lows, at the risk of future complications? If you are Type 1, are you interested in injections or a pump? If you are Type 2, would you prefer to try lifestyle change before medication? Do you prefer a doctor who speaks in technical terms, or one who breaks down information into simplistic terminology? Do you want a doctor who is easy-going and accepting, or one who will hold you accountable to taking care of yourself? Only you can determine the answers to those questions, as you are the one who has to live with diabetes. For example, I have decided to aim for normal BG and HgbA1C levels, at the risk of lows; I want to use a pump instead of injections; I prefer a doctor to speak to me in more technical terms due to my experience; and I prefer my doctor take my care seriously, even if it means holding me accountable. Finally, be aware that you may not find a doctor that meets *all* of your criteria, so you need to decide which areas you are willing to sacrifice.

Once you have developed your goals, you are ready to begin your search. While the occasional general practitioner is knowledgeable enough to help you, it is usually preferable to find an endocrinologist specializing in your type of diabetes. Don't just expect a doctor to be a diabetes expert. Doctors are not educated the same way. General practitioners, for example, have a good, overall understanding of how the body works, but not necessarily a specialized, focused understanding of specific areas of the body. An endocrinologist, on the other hand, specializes in the endocrine system. However, because the endocrine system has so many functions within the body, there are specialties within that system. So, ideally, you will seek out an endocrinologist specializing in your type of diabetes. Among diabetes specialists, most have a clientele consisting primarily of Type 2 diabetics. Many, if not the majority, of diabetics are considered "non-compliant," meaning they are either uninformed, in denial, or just opposed to making changes. As a result, many doctors aren't as concerned as they would be if they thought the patient wanted to improve, even if that meant sacrifice. If you are a Type 1, make sure the doctor also has large numbers of Type 1 diabetic patients. Despite what type of diabetes you have, or who you choose as a practitioner, be prepared to "prove" yourself in order to get the doctor's full cooperation. Don't limit your search to your local area. Many diabetics, myself included, have commuted several hours one way to find the best possible care.

When searching for a doctor, I recommend asking your doctor or his staff a few questions to find out what his specialty is. If you already have a doctor, you can ask around at your next appointment. You can also consider your past experiences with him. If you are still searching for a doctor, you can call different offices and ask questions over the phone. Most are happy to answer. Some may prefer a consult, so be prepared with an answer. Find out if the doctor works alone, or if he works alongside a diabetes educator and/or a diabetes nutritionist. The latter two can be wonderful resources to aid in your desire for diabetes control. Ask for an estimated number of patients with your type of diabetes. If you are on an insulin pump, or hope to be, then ask for an estimated number of patients who use pumps. Ask the doctor what his preferred BG targets are and why. Ask what his preferred Hemoglobin A1C targets are and why. Consider his personality and how he relates to you and your child, if applicable.

Use the information you gather to help you make a decision on whom you choose as a doctor. If your preferred doctor doesn't accept your insurance plan, ask about payment plans or cash discounts. Many offices offer these options. When you think you know which doctor you would like to try, ask how he/she prefers you to record your data. Every doctor is different. Finally, try out the doctor you choose for a short time. If you are a Type 2, ask the doctor his opinion regarding your odds of coming off medication. If you are not yet insulin dependent, and he says, "None," find out the reasoning. Although it is hotly debated among the medical profession, I know of a number of cases where people eliminated all their symptoms with the proper treatments and life changes. Remember, unlike Type 1, Type 2 diabetes is a progressive disease that can usually be stopped or even reversed *if* the necessary lifestyle changes are made early enough. Most specialists I have dealt with prefer to follow up with new patients at least once a month for several months, and then space visits to 2-4 times per year. Meet with the doctor 3-4 times (more if you feel comfortable, less if not) and do everything the doctor recommends. If, despite his recommendations, you are having trouble gaining or maintaining control of your blood sugars, you may want to consider trying another doctor. Though it may be inconvenient for a while, remember that your doctor is a partner in your health care. His recommendations, and your compatibility with him, can help determine how healthy you stay.

Finally, keep in mind that your doctor is only human. He or she may make mistakes, may have a bad day, and may advise you incorrectly on occasion. They are not perfect. Also, you must be willing to take control of your own disease. The doctor can give you the best advice available, but you must put it to use to help yourself. If your doctor gives you advice that you believe to be incorrect or dangerous, don't hesitate to ask him for reasoning. You are ultimately responsible for decisions about your body. Recently, I had a doctor who, for months, delayed signing paperwork for my records. This resulted in a lengthy delay for my insurance authorizations, which, in turn, could have caused a great deal of trouble if my prescriptions had expired. Because I had taken control of my situation, however, I was aware of this issue and was able to make the necessary arrangements with another doctor before a problem arose.

I mentioned previously how many diabetics are considered non-compliant. In my experience, when I walk into my appointment, fully prepared with 2-3 weeks worth of charts, graphs, logs, and data, recent lab work, as well as my written list of questions, the doctor instantly realizes that I am serious about controlling my diabetes, and I expect him or her to be also. The more effort you put into caring for yourself, and the better prepared you can be, the easier it is to be taken seriously. I guarantee you will stand out from your peers. I once had a doctor who would spend 45 minutes with me to tweak any detail I needed for control, while the average patient got 15 minutes. Because she saw I was serious, she truly wanted to help.

In addition to finding a good doctor, whom you trust with your life (literally), you may need to make some lifestyle changes. To put it simply and bluntly, *you* must decide whether you want to live or die. In order to live a healthy, happy, long life, free of complications, you may have to make some big changes. If you don't make the decision, and just take things as they come, you will inadvertently set yourself up for possible complications and even death much sooner than necessary. There are people who have been diabetic for over 50 years with no signs of complications, and others who have faced amputations or blindness after only two or three years. Unfortunately, many diabetics, Type 1's and Type 2's, show some type of complications within just a few years. However, in most cases, this is only because they didn't make the necessary lifestyle changes to control their disease. Even something as "simple" as short-term memory loss, often misdiagnosed as aging or dementia, may in fact, be a complication of diabetes.

Many factors influence your insulin requirements and blood sugars. While some factors are out of your control, you are directly responsible for others. For example, the more active you are, the less insulin you need. If you eat the wrong foods, you may set yourself up for high BGs afterwards. If you don't test frequently enough, there is no way to control your diabetes properly. For Type 1's, many doctors recommend testing four times a day, while others recommend 6. I have found 6-8 times works best for me, though I may do less on "good" days and more on "bad" days. It is unfortunate that many Type 2's are told to test only once per day, if that. You can't possibly know how your blood sugars are doing, unless you test regularly. As soon as possible, start getting to know your body better than you ever thought possible. Tell your doctor how many times per day you would like to test. Most doctors will be happy to write you a prescription if they think you are serious. If they try to discourage you, again, ask for reasoning. Record your blood sugars and insulin intake. There are software programs available that make this process much easier. Watch for patterns in your blood sugars which will help you determine how your body reacts to different influences such as food and activity. The more you learn about yourself, the easier controlling your diabetes becomes.

Concerning other factors that affect your BG levels, you need to become educated and aware so you can handle situations as they arise. Basically, these factors affect glucose levels in the blood by changing the body's level of resistance or sensitivity to insulin and its ease of absorption of glucose from the blood. Activity may affect your BG levels for some time after the activity has ended. Hormones can have a major influence on BGs. Males generally experience the most difficulty with hormone-related BG levels around the time of growth spurts and puberty, since their hormones generally stabilize afterward. Females, however, will deal with changing hormones on a regular basis, beginning with growth spurts and puberty, and continuing through menopause. Pregnancy can cause drastic changes to BG levels very rapidly. Like hormones, illness can cause BG changes. Different foods will affect levels, as wells as the amount of food eaten. Certain types of stress can affect levels, as can emotion to a certain extent. Excess weight has the effect of increased insulin resistance, as described previously. Drugs, including prescription medications, and alcohol can affect BG levels, and should generally be avoided whenever possible. While there are other factors that can affect BG levels, these are probably the easiest to prevent, monitor, and prepare for. I will go into more detail about each factor; however, I recommend you consult a more in-depth resource for additional information.

Activity

Activity, or a lack thereof, can have a tremendous affect on BG levels. Depending on your body, levels may be affected for only a short time, or for as long as a couple of weeks afterward. While there are many details involved, I have found this process easiest to understand by relating it to metabolism. Just like regular exercise can increase the efficiency of the body's use of food, activity also directly affects the body's use of insulin. The effect of exercise, however, is dependent on how much time and effort is involved. As a result, if you have a rather sedate, inactive lifestyle, such as sitting at a desk, in a car, or watching TV most of the day, you will require higher doses of insulin in order to absorb glucose from the blood. On the other hand, if you are a triathlete, participating in strenuous activity on a regular basis, then your cells will be more sensitive to glucose absorption, and little insulin will be required. I actually knew of one lady who was a Type 1 and a great example of the latter. Due to her physically active lifestyle and healthy eating habits, she required no basal rate of insulin on an average day. She only took a bolus when she ate. Chances are you fall somewhere in between, and, as a result, you must continually balance your insulin rates according to your activity level.

You should consult with your doctor about how best to calculate this balance. The best way to get started is to test regularly and document carefully for a while. Keep close records of activity types, and even develop a rating of intensity to help you keep track. Record durations of activity, and then record your BGs for the next 48 hours. Over time, you will begin to see patterns. I have found that going jogging for 15 minutes will affect me differently than trail riding my horse for 15 minutes, which will be different than riding my horse in the arena for 15 minutes. Likewise, gardening will have a different affect on my BGs than bicycling or cleaning house for a similar amount of time. A one-time activity session can easily affect your BG levels for up to 48 hours. Regular exercise, on the other hand, such as jogging every day for ½ hour, will likely cause an overall decrease in insulin requirements. If you then stop exercising temporarily, this effect can last up to a couple of weeks before you will have to increase your insulin. In either case, the activity can potentially cause a slight increase in your BG level around the time of the activity session. If your BG level is within a normal range, you will likely not notice this increase. If, however, your BG level is high, the stress hormones released during this activity will likely cause your level to increase noticeably.

Once you have discovered your patterns, you and your doctor will be better able to develop a plan. If you are on pills or injections, you may need to decrease your dosage for all or part of the day. If you are on a pump, you can figure out how much you should decrease your basal rate, and for how long. Keep in mind that because activity can influence you long after the activity itself has ended, you may find yourself experiencing low BGs in the middle of the night or the next day. It is all related. Your cells become very sensitive for a while and absorb glucose very easily, potentially causing these hypoglycemic reactions. Note that it is easiest to plan and control your BG levels with activity if you can manage a routine. For example, if you can schedule a 15 minute jog beginning at 7 a.m. every morning, then it will be much easier to predict and manage resulting lows, as compared to walking one morning, jogging the next evening, and doing nothing the third day.

Hormones

Hormones have many different life-sustaining functions and contributions. They are, in some part, responsible for growth, energy, digestion, muscle and hair development, and much more. They are also responsible for our "fight-or-flight" response. When you experience a low blood sugar, you may feel sweaty and shaky, which is due primarily to the "fight" hormones being released to defend your body against the danger of getting too low. Hormones can affect BG levels differently, and different people are affected by the same hormones in different ways. The only way to figure out how your hormones affect your BG levels, once again, is to test regularly and record carefully. Look for patterns over the course of time and around certain events. This information will help you and your doctor develop a plan for controlling BGs. For more detailed information regarding female hormones and pregnancy, see the chapter "Just For Diabetic Women."

Illness

Oh, don't you dread those sick days? It just so happens, however, that you can use diabetes to your advantage in this case! By becoming familiar with patterns of BG levels, you may notice a slight rise in your BG levels 24 hours or even several days prior to feeling the first symptom of an illness. With many colds and illnesses, as well as some invasive injuries, the combination of a decrease in activity and the natural illness-fighting defense responses of your body results in an increase in BG levels. You may require more insulin to stabilize your BG levels while you are sick. Once you know your patterns, you and your doctor can develop a system of increasing your insulin at the onset of an illness, before your BGs increase too much.

Food

Food is an area that seems to confuse many people, not limited to diabetics. Most people today walk to their cupboard or fridge, grab a bite to eat, and never give a moments thought as to how the body handles that food. As a diabetic, you need to be aware if you want to be in control of your BG levels.

Diabetics are generally most concerned about their starch, or carbohydrate, intake. The majority of foods contain carbohydrates in some level, including dairy, vegetables, fruits, some fats, and meats, as well as most drinks. Some foods, such as fats, meat, and most vegetables, contain levels minute enough that most doctors don't acknowledge them. For veggies, a good rule of thumb is to taste it. Sweet vegetables such as peas, corn, sweet potatoes, and even carrots likely contain enough sugars that you should count them as carbohydrates. Non-sweet veggies such as lettuce, asparagus, eggplant, and tomatoes, you likely won't count in your carb intake due to the minute levels they contain.

There are two ways to calculate your carbohydrate intake, and it often depends on whether you use diet, pills, insulin injections, or a pump. One way is the method that is most familiar and found on the Food Guide Pyramid provided by the USDA. It suggests eating 6-11 servings of carbohydrates each day. Many diabetics who use pills and injections base their doses on the assumption that a particular number of servings will be consumed each day. Consuming less than that number will result in low blood sugars (because the pills or insulin is in the system, but not the food), while consuming more will result in high blood sugars (because the glucose is in the system, but not the meds).

The second method, often used by pumpers or users of short-acting insulin, is a carb-counting method. With this system, rather than counting servings, you count the estimated grams of carbohydrates being consumed, and take insulin according to the actual carb consumption. The easiest way to understand the difference between these two methods is to look at a food label. The label on a box of cereal may state the serving size as one half cup, which would be the equivalent of one carbohydrate serving for the day. Further down on the label, however, it may state, "Total Carbohydrates, 30 grams" in that half cup serving (see Figure 1). Talk to your doctor about which method is best for you.

Figure 1:

→

Nutrition Facts	
Serving Size ½ cup (33g)	
Servings Per Container 15	

Amount Per Serving	
Calories 100	

	% Daily Value*
Total Fat 3g	22%
Sodium 6 mg	40%
Total Carbohydrate 30g	12%
Sugars 25g	
Protein 9g	18%

*Percent Daily Values are based on a 2,000 calorie diet.

→ (appears next to the Total Carbohydrate row)

I highly recommend learning to read food labels, as they are a storehouse of information. You will likely be amazed how one small package of crackers, may in fact be two and a half servings of carbohydrates. Likewise, plain roasted peanuts may have five grams of carbs in 40 peanuts; while honey-roasted or candy-coated peanuts are one carb per peanut. Since learning to read labels, I have become quite particular about what I eat, and how much. When it comes to juice, I only drink 100% juice. Literally, the ingredients are juice, water, and ascorbic (or citric) acid. By eliminating fillers and additives, these companies also cut sugar content by significant amounts. A great rule of thumb I once heard for improving your diet based on food labels was to avoid any food that contained an ingredient you couldn't pronounce! To take it a step further, a friend of mine summarized this with the rule of thumb to, "shop around the edge of the grocery store; that covers your produce, meat, dairy, and bread. Everything in the aisles is likely full of chemicals and sugar!" My family tries to go as natural and organic as possible, based on the availability of supplies in our area. Remember, however, that organic means free of chemicals, and doesn't necessarily mean healthy. Organic junk food does exist, and many organic foods are loaded with natural sugars and carbs.

Once you understand how to calculate your carb intake, then you must understand how food is absorbed by the body. The moment food enters your mouth, your saliva begins the digestive process, and sugars are absorbed by the mouth into the bloodstream. There are two types of carbohydrates, or sugars—simple and complex. Simple sugars are absorbed faster than complex sugars, because the complex sugars must be broken down more, which takes time. Simple sugars are usually found in anything made with fruit, white or brown sugar, white flours, or natural sugars such as honey and syrup. Juices and most sugary drinks are simple as well. Simple sugars are generally absorbed by the bloodstream very quickly, and therefore, insulin must be taken in advance of consumption. Complex sugars are usually found in foods made with whole grains. Other foods can also affect the way carbohydrates are absorbed. Fats, protein, and fiber, for example, can slow absorption. For example, pizza, which is made of white flour and sugar, and would normally be considered a simple carb, also contains oils and proteins that delay absorption of the sugars as if they were more complex. For more information, read the chapter, "Good Food, Bad Food."

Based on the above, if you are having an issue with low blood sugars, you want to take simple sugars to get your blood sugar up fast. If you are having a problem with high blood sugars, particularly after a meal, you may want to focus more on complex carbs, proteins, and fiber. In either case, when you must eat simple sugars, then consider adding plenty of protein, fats, and/or fiber to the meal to slow the absorption somewhat and help stabilize the BG levels.

In regards to low blood sugar, there is an appropriate way to treat it. Understandably, simple sugars are preferable because of their fast rate of absorption. Additionally, the less digesting that needs to occur, the faster the sugar will be absorbed. For example, sugar water or 100% juice will be absorbed faster than soda, which will be absorbed faster than a cookie. Once you decide what to treat with, then figure out how much to treat with. If you find that a full cup of juice makes your BG go from 55 to 150 in 15 minutes, then you may want to try one half cup of juice next time. I count grams of carbs, and my treatment of choice is juice boxes due to their portability and convenience. They also come in a selection of sizes, most commonly 15 grams of carbs and 24 grams. I have found that, without insulin, 10 grams of carbs will increase my BG level about 25 points when I am low. So if my BG falls to 65, I drink about 10 carbs worth of juice to reach my preferred target of 90. If my BG is 40, then I need to drink about 20 carbs worth to reach a BG of 90. If you find hunger is a symptom of your lows, then treat the low as needed, and munch on items like carrots, cheese, or celery to fulfill your desire to eat. Consuming more carbs than necessary when you treat a low not only risks a high BG shortly after, but also results in the consumption of extra, unnecessary calories. Talk with your doctor, monitor your current techniques, and calculate exactly how many carbs you need to increase your BG to your desired level.

Whether diabetic or not, most people find they have the "munchies" at some point. While the majority of people only have to worry about weight gain, diabetics must worry about weight as well as glucose levels and carb intake. For these occasions, I recommend forming a list of foods you and your doctor consider acceptable for those cravings. My "munchie" of choice is actually not even a food. I tend to chew gum. Most of the time when I feel the need to snack, I am not truly hungry; rather, I simply want something in my mouth. As long as I chew a sugarless gum, I don't have to worry about insulin. Other foods on my "acceptable" list include beef jerky (again, for the chew factor), unsweetened trail mix, and vegetables. Only when my sugars are stabilized in a healthy range do I allow myself to splurge on something that requires insulin to counteract it.

Speaking of splurging, most people splurge on occasion, be it at the Sunday buffet, a dinner party, or just a midnight craving. Some splurges may involve healthy food in excess, while others may involve pure "junk" and sweet deserts. While I know it isn't a healthy thing to do, I am as guilty as anybody. To handle these situations, I have become aware of how my body handles different foods, and I have developed a list of "rules" that I discipline myself to follow. I mentioned eating too much of healthy foods, and by that I mean that the body actually reacts just to the fact that the stomach is full, regardless of whether it is full of celery or cake. There is a lot of physiological detail involved in this situation that goes beyond the scope of this book and can be found in other resources, so I will not go into detail here. Just be aware that, due to the body's natural responses to a full stomach, over-eating will likely result in a high blood sugar several hours after the meal. In addition, you may experience low BGs shortly after the meal. You can avoid this difficult-to-control response by not eating any more once you are *satisfied*.

I have learned that my body doesn't handle overeating well at all. It never fails that I will experience a low about 30 minutes to an hour after the meal (due to the bolus of insulin I took). Then, about four hours after the large meal, my BG will hit around 300 if I don't monitor closely. Additionally, there are some foods such as pizza and pasta that I cannot eat more than about a half of a serving, or I will have unstable BGs for up to 24 hours afterward.

Splurging on sweets is another issue. As unhealthy as it is, I admit I have a sweet tooth! To deal with my desire for sweets, I moderate as best I can. For example, I won't allow myself to eat "junk" cereals, and if I do eat a honey-covered or high-carb cereal such as granola, then I usually mix it with a healthier, lower-carb cereal. If I want to splurge on the assortment of desserts at a party, then I severely limit the amount of carbs I eat during the main course. Furthermore, I ensure my BGs are stable and around my target range before I splurge. There are times where I take more drastic measures. For example, there is a brunch restaurant in my town that my family loves. However, I tend to eat too many carbs every time we visit there, which results in high BG levels for the rest of the day. We have decided to avoid this restaurant completely, as a result. My recommendation to you is to decide what is most important and/or enjoyable for you *before* the fact. Work with your doctor to develop a plan, and discipline yourself to stick with it. If necessary, ask someone to hold you accountable (but don't be offended if they do!)

Healthy eating may be something you already do and will therefore come easily. If not, this step may be more difficult. If you are the latter, consider the two following things:

1. The first two weeks of a new lifestyle are the hardest. If you can make it through 14 days, just taking it one day at a time, it *will* get easier!

2. A new, healthier lifestyle and eating habits will improve your whole family's health. If you are reading this in order to help a loved one with diabetes, realize that changing bad habits is one of the most difficult things to do. This is no exception for a diabetic. Therefore, one of the most meaningful steps you can take to support the lifestyle they need to have, is to make a few changes yourself. It could literally mean the difference in them having severe complications within 10 years, or living a healthy, complication-free life for 50 or more years

Just commit to change, throw out the junk food, and only buy what you should. Remember, if junk isn't in the house and convenient, you will be less likely to eat it.

Stress

Another hotly debated topic in the medical profession is whether stress influences blood glucose values. However, I and many of the diabetics I know have noticed certain stress-related factors seem to play a very big role in our BG levels. Based on our experiences and what I have gathered from doctors and research over the years, I would sum the stress factor up as follows:

The stress that most people think of when we hear the term is the long-term, chronic type caused by work, school, family, or other factors. This type of stress can be intense and long-lasting, but interestingly, has little, if any, affect on BG levels. When BGs are affected, it is more likely related to a lack of activity or an increase in eating resulting from the stress. There is another type of stress which can affect BGs. It is a short-term stress and is caused by things like short-term anxiety, extreme excitement, and unusual, sudden fear. All of these emotions can cause a release of hormones and/or a use of energy that increases or decreases a cell's ability to absorb glucose from the blood stream. This, in turn, can cause high or low BG levels. A good example is a child who is excited about going to Disneyland or an adult anxious about giving a speech to a large group. In either case, there is likely to be an affect on BG levels. If I have a presentation to give to an audience, I must carefully monitor my BG levels for several hours prior to the event, and I often eat a small protein-based snack just beforehand to prevent a low from the anxiety I often experience. However, every body is different, and you must determine how your body is affected in order to develop a plan to prevent or prepare for these fluctuations.

Another stress most people are unaware of is exercise. As I detailed in the "Activity" section, exercise will very likely stress the body just enough to increase the BG level in the short term. So, if you are already experiencing a high sugar level, hold off until you know the BG level is returning to normal.

Circadian Rhythm

Your body is on a natural "time-clock," called the circadian rhythm. This process is partly responsible for your feelings of wakefulness and your desire for sleep. While this rhythm can be trained to an extent (i.e. a night-shift worker vs. a day-shift worker), different studies and examples over the years have found the rhythm to be on a 24-hour clock. You may have heard about prisoners and test subjects who have had no way to tell time quickly get a cycle that often corresponds with natural sunlight and darkness.

As a part of this rhythm, your body functions work differently during different times of the day. For example, some functions such as digestion tend to slow down during the sleep hours, then pick up again shortly before breakfast, which causes the hungry feeling you experience when you awake. Hormonal releases vary throughout the day. As a result of these changing rhythms, blood sugars can be affected. If you are not a schedule-oriented person, circadian-rhythm-related BG changes can be harder to predict. However, if you generally wake at the same time each morning, eat at similar times, and go to bed at a similar time each night, your rhythm becomes very predictable. In turn, your BG patterns become more predictable.

You may have noticed that weekends (or days off work), as well as times of travel, have a drastic affect on your BG levels. This is due to the fact that the natural body rhythms have been thrown out of whack. Most people tend to sleep late on weekends, or have a different routine on days off. An example is how diet on weekends is often different than weekdays. You may have an insulin rate set according to drinking a quick shake for breakfast, and then a simple lunch. On weekends, however, perhaps you eat eggs and pancakes for breakfast, snack on potato chips while watching Saturday-morning cartoons, then have some leftovers for lunch and dinner. Chances are you consume more carbs than you are used to, and this may throw off your BG levels. You could work with your doctor to develop a possible insulin regimen for weekdays, and a different one for weekends.

You may have a totally different lifestyle while traveling. Traveling may also add time change to the mix of factors, throwing off your rhythm even further. You can prepare to some extent for these changes by testing regularly, finding patterns in your records, and working with your doctor to develop a plan for your insulin regimen. There are two ways to handle time changes, depending on whether the travel is short-term or long-term.

For short-term time changes, you can either keep your routine on your time, despite what the local time is. For example, let's assume you live in Pacific Standard Time, and wake at 7 a.m. each morning. If you travel to the East Coast for a few days, then you could simply get up at 10 a.m. Of course, time changes don't always work out this way.

The other option, best suited for long term travel (longer than one week) is to immediately put your body on the "local" time, and gradually change the time for your meds or insulin. For example, when I travel to a location two hours ahead for less than three days, I actually leave my pump time set as my original location since my circadian rhythm is on the original time. However, if the trip is longer than three days, then my rhythm will begin to shift to the new time. Around day three, I will change my pump clock by one hour, then about two days later, turn it closer to the local time by another hour. This helps my insulin keep up with the new rhythm being set in my body. My husband is a military pilot. He has told me how, in his training, it was emphasized that the best way to be alert when changing time zones (such as a deployment) was to force himself to go to bed at the "local" bedtime, wake with the "local" sunrise, and stick to your normal routine using the local time. For example, he generally awakes at 6 a.m., exercises, eats a hearty breakfast, and so on, until he goes to bed at 10 p.m. When he travels to a different time zone, he will stay awake (if necessary) so he can go to bed at 10 pm local time. He then gets up at 6 a.m. local time, and starts his routine from there. He is generally able to get over jet-lag within 24 hours, and get his body on schedule by keeping his morning and bedtime routines the same, but always being on the local time— even if the local time was EST in the morning and somewhere half way around the world at bedtime and the next morning.

Dawn Phenomenon

A term you will likely hear often is "dawn phenomenon." It goes hand-in-hand with the circadian rhythm, and is generally to blame for unexplained high blood sugars before breakfast. This is caused by a complicated process in which the liver basically prepares the body for the daily carb intake by removing glucose already in the blood stream. The sudden decrease in blood glucose causes a secondary response involving the release of glucose back into the blood stream. While this same process may occur in a non-diabetic, they also produce insulin to counteract the glucose. A diabetic lacks that insulin, though, which results in a high BG value. This is rather complex process that is beyond the scope of this book. You can find more detailed information in other sources, but you should be aware of the basics at least. Although the dawn phenomenon is not usually dangerous, the high BG levels it causes can be frustrating. The problem can be solved by becoming familiar with your body's patterns, and then your doctor can advise accordingly using diet and insulin appropriately to counter the effect.

Drugs and Alcohol

All substances can potentially have an affect on the body, and in the case of a diabetic, on blood sugar levels. When your doctor prescribes medicine, he is usually aware of the affect the medication can have on the insulin resistance. There are some medications which, as a general rule, are not prescribed to diabetics. There are others that have enough of an affect you will have to increase or decrease your pill dosage or basal insulin rate to some extent. There are others that will have little to no affect on BG levels. Many over-the-counter medicines contain sugars which require insulin just like food. Although doctors and pharmacists are typically cautious and aware of what is being prescribed, I recommend you always ask. Mistakes do happen. I specifically ask my doctor if there are any known affects on BG levels, and then I tend to double-check with the pharmacist when I pick up the meds. There have been several occasions where my doctor just forgot to mention the effects, but because I asked, I was able to prepare accordingly.

Illegal drugs and abuse of legal drugs can be extra lethal to a diabetic, and should be avoided at all costs. Because you are probably already aware of the dangers generally associated with these drugs, I won't go into detail. However, I will leave you with the two following scenarios: First, imagine taking a drug such as a depressant or narcotic, which slows down bodily functions. Let's assume you pass out or black out for a while. During that time, you have a very low blood sugar. You would be unable to treat it, which could potentially result in permanent brain damage or death. On the other hand, let's say you took a stimulant or hallucinogen. Because these drugs commonly cause reactions such as shaking, hallucinations, confusion, and more, again, you may not realize you are having a low. Even if you do, you may not have the cognitive ability to treat the low.

Similarly, alcohol is a depressant, and some drinks can be high in calories and carbs. The latter can have a major impact on blood sugar levels. Furthermore, many diabetics who were known to drink have been mistakenly assumed to be drunk and, therefore, ignored as they experienced a low blood sugar reaction requiring assistance.

Diabetes has enough risks in itself. It is also hard enough to stay in control of your disease and to properly care for yourself with normal, day-to-day influences. There is just no justifiable reason to add the additional factors of illegal drugs, abusing legal drugs, or alcohol to the situation. Although I have heard people argue that a glass of wine every day can be beneficial, there are many other dietary things you can change and get the same benefit. In the long run, you will be thankful you avoided it.

Body Conditioning

I am not referring to exercise when I refer to body conditioning here. I am, instead, referring to the fact that you can condition your body to accept the abnormal as normal. A person who loves fast food and hates vegetables has conditioned their body that way. Similarly, a person who routinely has BGs around 200, and feels OK, has conditioned their body to accept that level as normal, and therefore, may feel symptoms of a low when their BG level is 100. If the body becomes conditioned to accept high BGs as normal, that basically means that the body is sustaining high enough sugars to cause long-term damage and complications. On the opposite extreme, a person who has frequent low blood sugars may condition their body to accept a 50 as normal. The body is designed to react to low BGs by exhibiting low BG symptoms. Normally, symptoms should start around 75-80. However, if the body accepts 50 as normal, then no symptoms will be felt until the BG reaches 45 or lower. Obviously, this could easily result in seizure or even death.

Fortunately, the body can be reconditioned. Reconditioning is difficult and uncomfortable for a while, due to the symptoms experienced. For example, if your BG runs high, you may be weak, shaky, and hungry as though you are very low, when in fact, your sugar is 120. However, it is certainly healthier to deal with this temporary discomfort in order to improve your overall well-being. The key to reconditioning your body is do it gradually, over days, weeks, or even a month or two, depending on the degree of change necessary. It took me eight months to learn to enjoy vegetables after marrying my health-conscious husband, but now I crave them if I go a day without. Ask your doctor's advice for a target BG range, and wean yourself to it.

Dehydration

Doctors differ on their opinions of this issue, but in my experience, dehydration can have an effect on blood sugars. Most of the time, it seems to cause high blood sugars. However, just because your BG level may be low does not necessarily mean you aren't dehydrated. It is proven that dehydration causes many issues, including, but not necessarily limited to, vision changes, headaches, fatigue, drowsiness, and more. So it only makes sense that it can affect BG concentration levels. One good way to tell if you are dehydrated is to check the color of your urine. The clearer your urine, the more hydrated you are. To the contrary, the more yellow it is, the more dehydrated you are. If you have any doubt, drink a glass of water and test your sugar!

Medical Situations

As a diabetic, you need to have a "hospital plan." As much as possible, this plan should include everything from an unexpected trip to the Emergency Room to a scheduled surgery or overnight stay. Unfortunately, not all medical personnel are knowledgeable about diabetes, and many welcome knowledge and information regarding how best to care for your diabetes while you are in their care. You should consider wearing a medical alert bracelet or some other way of being easily identified as a diabetic. You can write down all sorts of information about your health status, history, and physician contact information on a card that is stored with your driver's license. Finally, you should have a list of needed supplies somewhere at home where a loved one can easily access it in the event you need someone to bring them to you. If you use a pump, be aware that few nurses and doctors have training with pumps. Therefore, in most cases, if you are unable to care for yourself, they will try to remove the pump and put you on injections or intravenous insulin for the duration of your stay. You should be prepared for this situation. (See "Appendix E" for ideas).

I learned the importance of planning and preparing for hospital situations with my pregnancies. With my first pregnancy, my complications were very sudden and unexpected. When I was 32 weeks, I went to a routine appointment, and within minutes of being examined, the doctor discovered I was in pre-term labor. My contractions were already three minutes apart. He ordered me to go straight to the hospital Labor and Delivery Ward. I didn't get out until a week later. Fortunately, my husband had been assisting me with my pump for a few weeks since my growing belly was making it difficult to insert my infusion sites alone. As a result, he had learned what I needed. He was able to go home and pack my medical supplies into a hospital bag for me. After I was released from the hospital, I gave him some additional lessons on my pump and reviewed all the settings and pump functions. The effort quickly paid off. When the time came for me to deliver, due to a long series of events (not related to my diabetes), I had to have an emergency c-section. While they prepped me, I actually passed out and remained unconscious throughout the surgery, and for a total of about four hours. During that time, the doctor used my husband's knowledge of my care. The staff tested my BG level regularly throughout the early part of the ordeal, but at one point, the hospital meter gave inconsistent readings. The doctor had my husband test me, using my meter, and used that value to make decisions. He had my husband remove my pump site to prevent an accidental overdose of insulin. After the surgery (and after getting my husband's permission), the doctor ordered the nurses to allow my husband to control my insulin and BG monitoring until I regained consciousness. My husband inserted a fresh infusion site, and programmed my pump based on his knowledge and the doctor's calculations, and the staff in the delivery ward were very respectful and cooperative with my husband's requests. After the ordeal, I woke up in much better shape than when it all began! I also woke up 25 pounds lighter! Our planning and preparations certainly paid off during that ordeal!

Learn to Cope

Learning how to cope emotionally with a new diagnosis can be just as difficult as learning to cope physically. I have known people who received their diagnosis, then basically gave up on life. They allowed their disease to take control of their body, and suffered complications in a short amount of time. I have known others who received their diagnosis, then determined that life would go on. You must learn to do both if you are going to take control of your disease.

People have asked me how I cope. Honestly, I think it would be difficult to do without my personal belief in Jesus Christ. I have experienced some tough times, some of which were quite frightening. He was the source I would turn to for peace. Over the years, I have realized that there are many other diseases or conditions I could have that are much worse than diabetes. With diabetes, I could essentially determine how healthy I wanted to be based on how attentive I was to my disease. I noticed that the more I learned about controlling it, the more habitual my actions became, and BG control was easier.

I will note that many newly diagnosed diabetics talk about their disease more than they realize. It is only natural, as suddenly this condition has intruded into your life and seemingly taken over every thought you posses. Other people's reactions to your conversation may vary. Those who are closest to you will be curious and concerned for a while, but their interest will decrease over time. Some people may want to ask you questions, but be nervous that they will offend you or make you uncomfortable. Others will be uncomfortable with the topic, and would prefer to treat you the way they did before the diagnosis. Still others simply don't care. While it is understandable for you to mention it shortly after your diagnosis, if you are not careful, you can easily alienate yourself from your friends and acquaintances by discussing your diabetes too much. If you feel a great need to talk about how you feel, and you think it would help you cope, there are other ways. You can talk to a pastor, a close confidant (but use caution not to wear out your welcome!), or even find new diabetic friends in the same situation. Your local hospital or an internet search may help you find a wide selection of diabetes support groups, chat rooms, classes, and programs.

However you choose to cope, there will come a point that you must just accept what you have, accept the lifestyle changes that go along with it, and move on. You may try to distract yourself by getting involved in a hobby. Just be careful not to get so involved that you forget to be attentive to your health. If you find yourself becoming depressed, you should seek professional counsel. Depression will only make it more difficult to take control of your diabetes. Fact is, you are not the only person to have ever experienced this. Remember, there are millions of diabetics around the world, and most have experienced what you are going through right now.

Finally, realize that it *will* get easier. Like any new thing, you must focus on your new condition and learn about it at first. The more you learn however, and the more involved you become in your medical care, the faster it will become second nature. Soon, it will become comforting to test your BG level, and you will do it almost automatically anytime you don't feel right. At this point, I can test my BG level in bed, in the dark, without disturbing my sleeping husband. I can calculate my insulin boluses just by looking at a plate of food. It will happen, but you must put forth the effort to learn in the beginning.

Learn to Live

Finally, once you have figured out how different factors affect your body and your BG levels, learn how to live and enjoy life. I do recommend you set some standards for yourself. Though some may require some self-discipline, sacrifice, or inconvenience, it will help you be your best. For example, decide on a BG level that you must be above to drive. If, at any time while driving, you sense a possible drop in BG level, commit yourself to pull over immediately and test. Stopping on the side of the road for two minutes is worth it to prevent a major accident. While I normally wouldn't treat a BG level higher than 75, if I am going to drive, I might eat a small amount of carbs at a BG of 80. This is an important step toward being a responsible diabetic driver and preventing accidents.

Develop plans for situations that could *potentially* turn into emergencies. For example, if you accidentally administer too much insulin, have someone you can call and agree to a time within two hours or so when you will call back. That way, if you don't call again, they know to check on you. I remember a time when I was home alone and mistakenly injected insulin into a vein. Within seconds, I actually felt my BG level dropping. I quickly grabbed the phone, called my husband, and told him what had happened. I told him I was going to test my BG level for the next 15 minutes and call him back. Fortunately, I had injected only a small amount of insulin (about a half unit), so my BG level only dropped to about 70. However, should this situation have gotten worse, my husband was aware and prepared to call for help if he didn't hear back from me.

When you do go out alone, ensure you have not only your test kit, but also a spare syringe and insulin, low BG treatments, and some spare cash. It is always a good idea to tell someone where you will be. I know of one situation where a guy didn't report home and it was two days before he was found unconscious in his vehicle from a severe low. Only God knows why he survived that long. Perhaps you should even keep a juice box and phone by your bed for nighttime emergencies. Another example is when we asked a few, close neighbors to be on standby in the event of a diabetic emergency. My husband leaves for work quite early, but will call me almost every morning, about half an hour after I get up. If I don't answer the phone and he can't leave, then he can call one of these neighbors to come check on me.

You can think up a few other preventative measures based on your particular lifestyle. After you do what you can to prepare, however, then relax and enjoy life.

4

Good Food, Bad Food

Since the subject of this book is to take control of your health, I thought it would be appropriate to add a short chapter devoted to food. You have probably heard the saying "you are what you eat." If you eat unhealthy foods, you are likely to be unhealthy. If you eat sweet foods, you will likely crave only sweets. On the other hand, if you eat well-balanced, wholesome foods, your body will function as God designed it to. There are so many books today devoted to the subject of eating healthy, you may be wondering why I would bother to even add this chapter.

Over the last few years, we have had several health situations arise in my family. My first son experienced seizures as an infant that seemed to be linked to our water source at the time. Later, he developed an ear infection. While being treated with antibiotics, he had a severe reaction to the penicillin. In order to help stop the reaction, his pediatrician recommended we allow him to eat and drink only organic dairy and meat products until all the antibiotic had been flushed from his system. About a year later, I developed severe hives that doctors could not explain. For months, I battled itching and welts until we stumbled upon some information about how preservatives in foods affect the body. As an experiment, we consumed a strictly organic diet for one week. Amazingly, my hives disappeared within 24 hours.

Those experiences, as well as a few others, made us curious as to what exactly we were putting into our bodies. We began asking questions and trying to make sense of these experiences. Why did my son need to eat only organic during his reaction? Why would organic foods clear up my hives? And, if foods could affect us in these ways, could foods also be affecting my diabetes? We began to research, reading and watching everything we could find. We were amazed to discover what was involved in the commercial food processing industry.

The dairy and meat industry must feed thousands of animals as cheaply as possible. These animals are housed in small, confined quarters, which can easily result in sickness and loss of profits. In order to help prevent these losses, the industry developed an antibiotic program to prevent illness in the animals. They also added hormones into the program to help the animals produce as much end product as possible. The problem is that these antibiotics and hormones spill over into the end product, which we consumers purchase from our local grocery store and then consume. Organic dairy and meat, on the other hand, must meet stricter regulations. Hormones and antibiotics cannot be administered, which keeps the food more natural. This explained why my son required organic during his reaction. The penicillin antibiotic he was prescribed for his ear infection was the same drug that is administered to many animals in the food chain. Because it was so crucial that he flush all the antibiotic from his system, giving him standard meat and dairy would have slowed this process.

Other processed foods are not much better, unfortunately. The commercial food industry must make a profit in order to stay in business. However, in order to produce a product as inexpensively as possible, they must ensure that they use as few expensive (natural) ingredients as possible, that the end product has a lengthy shelf life, and that it tastes good to the consumer who will purchase it. As a result, many companies use cheap, nutritionless fillers in the foods, unnatural, chemical preservatives are added to lengthen shelf life, and excessive amounts of sugar is added to increase palatability. These chemicals and preservatives had, apparently, built up in my system, resulting in the unexplained hives. As soon as I stopped consuming more, I allowed my body to purge itself of the toxins, and the hives disappeared.

Due to the discoveries we made during our research, we began to experiment with our diet. We began using a reverse osmosis system for our drinking water and drinking raw (unpasteurized, unhomogenized) milk from a trusted source. We began eating more produce, and, to reduce our pesticide intake, we purchased organic whenever possible. In order to reduce the amount of fillers and preservatives we ate, I began making as much as possible from scratch. I learned to bake crackers, yeast breads, cakes, pies, and many other baked goods. I started preserving produce at home, using non-chemical methods such as freezing, dehydrating, and canning. To reduce our processed sugar intake, I began used natural sweeteners in my cooking, such as honey, rapadura, and maple syrup, instead of processed white sugar. I also discovered Stevia, a wonderful, undigestable, natural sweetener that is perfect for a diabetic. In the event I did use processed sugars, I significantly reduced the amount the recipe called for. I incorporated plenty of whole grains and natural fiber into our diet. Interestingly, as we made these changes, we began to notice an overall improvement in our health. Our immunity improved drastically, and we rarely caught any type of virus. My migraines and headaches stopped. Chronic infections (which are known to be common in diabetics) went away. We felt better, had more energy, and experienced more refreshing sleep. Eventually, I noticed a change in my BG numbers. Although I still had occasional issues with high or low values, they were generally easy to explain. Overall, my BG levels were easier to stabilize, and fluctuated less.

Then I noticed an improvement in my lab panel. In fact, the day I had the appointment to get my improved lab results, the doctor was very rushed. She sent in an assistant, who I had never met, to discuss my results. He spent about 10 minutes looking over and telling me the results. As he finished, he pointed to a particular result and remarked, "This value seems slightly off to me. We may have to monitor it closely, as it could mean you have an increased risk of developing diabetes." I was stunned. My lab results had been so good, so *normal*, this assistant did not even realize I had been a Type 1 for 24 years! When I told him, he was speechless, and said he had never seen such results from a diabetic.

Now, more than ever, I am a big believer in the effects of diet and lifestyle. I encourage you to research the foods you are eating, talk to your doctor, and see if there are any changes you can make to improve your diet. The more natural and chemical-free your diet is, the better your body will function. While change can seem overwhelming, I learned, that if taken just one step at a time, it is much easier. For example, don't expect to just wake up one day and change everything. Rather, set some priorities. Change just one thing at a time. It may be one new thing a week or one a month. Then, enjoy witnessing your health and quality of life improve as you take control.

5

Just For Parents of Diabetic Children

If your child has recently been diagnosed with diabetes, you are probably fearing for his or her life right now, and wondering what you did wrong. First, let me assure you that *you did nothing wrong*. To the contrary, by getting a diagnosis, you have done things right! You recognized that something wasn't right with your child, you sought medical advice, and you got your child the attention he needed to survive! You are likely losing sleep as you try to prevent nighttime lows. If you have already witnessed the traumatic results of a severe hypoglycemic reaction, I can only imagine how frightened you must be. Realize that, although severe reactions are certainly dangerous, they are common among diabetics with unstable BG levels. Controlling diabetes, and thereby preventing reactions such as seizures, is a skill that must be studied and learned. That can take some time. Accept that you are going to make a few mistakes along the way. You can only do your best. Then understand that the body is a miraculous creation, and particularly with children, it has an amazing ability to heal and recover. Your child's age and level of maturity will determine his or her ability to comprehend what this new diagnosis means. While you are thinking of survival, thinking of the "what if's," and wondering what the future holds, chances are your child has other issues he is concerned with. Allow me to offer some tips and suggestions based on my personal experience and my encounters with other parents and children with diabetes, to help you and your child adapt.

Whether your child has Type 1 or Type 2, one of the first tips I can offer is to allow the diabetes management program recommended by your doctor to become an integrated part of your daily lifestyle. If you don't fight the changes needed, you will find control comes easier. One big way to do this is to go through your refrigerator and cupboards, and remove all sugary treats, cereals, snacks, and drinks. Give them away, or better yet, throw them away. If you are preaching to your child that sweets are bad, but then you eat cookies for snack, life will be very difficult. Young children will not understand why they can't eat what mommy, daddy, and siblings eat, and older children will simply begin to resent their disease to the point of rebelling.

The second tip I can offer is to be careful how often you blame your child's behavior on blood sugars. As an example, when I was a teen, if I got moody or depressed, my mom often asked "How have your sugars been today?" While the question itself is innocent and caring, sometimes your child may just want a hug, to talk, or just to be left alone. Whether or not fluctuating BG levels are to blame for your child's moods, the point is, they still have emotions that need care too. Older children may be perfectly aware that their fatigue and depression is related to their BG levels, however, pressuring them will most likely not help. Genuine concern and a loving shoulder to cry on may help your child get through the slump much faster, and will be more appreciated.

Finally, at some point, you may consider sending your child to a diabetes camp or support group. You should talk to your child's doctor and your child about this, and carefully consider their response. A younger child or tween-age may be very interested and even excited about joining such a group and getting involved with others "like them." A teen, on the other hand, may not want to participate in any group that reminds them of their disability. Rather, they usually want to be "like everyone else." If you feel your child should be part of some group, talk to your child and ask for their ideas and input. Listen carefully, as they may have an idea you would have never thought of. In the mean time, you may consider joining a support group yourself. Be aware that your child will likely learn a few "shortcuts" (aka cheating) in the management of their diabetes when attending these groups. I once spoke at a diabetes support group that involved refreshments consisting of sugary cookies, candies, fruit juices, and sodas. You should watch your child closely at such events. You could also be the parent that brings a healthy alternative such as a veggie or meat and cheese tray! Based on personal experience, I firmly believe that camps and support networks offer many advantages. Just be aware that your child may learn a few undesirable things from the other kids, in addition to the many good things they learn. Be prepared for this.

Once you have taken that first step, your child's age will determine what is needed from you, in addition to normal parental responsibilities.

Infant - Preschooler
Young children are worried about toys, playtimes, and why mommy and daddy are suddenly so attentive. This sudden, smothering attention can scare him a bit. To the contrary, it may backfire and result in a spoiled rotten child who always expects to be the center of attention. Be sure to continue allowing him to be a kid. Don't isolate him from playmates or discourage beloved activities, rather, learn how to prepare and take precautions for him.

When he is playing intently, he won't notice he doesn't feel good and that his blood sugar has dropped or increased until he is just too "sick" to keep playing. Once he complains to you, he will exhibit symptoms you will soon be very familiar with.

For a low sugar, he may be passive, sweaty, hungry, sleepy, or a combination of those symptoms and others. Most parents agree that the first thing they notice is a "glassy-eyed" or dazed appearance when they look in his eyes, or a pale look to their skin. Additionally, you may notice your child gets increasingly quiet and subdued. In any case, if you suspect a low sugar, test him. If he is low, encourage him to eat or drink some type of sugary item, in an amount pre-determined by your doctor. By limiting what your child consumes, you can prevent a rebounding high blood sugar that will cause a "roller-coaster" effect. Your child may be hungry for some time after a low, so talk with your doctor for recommendations. Foods like cheeses, lunch meats, vegetables, and other non-carb items are usually safe to eat in larger quantities without noticeable effects on blood sugar. Children can react differently, so you will learn if your child wants to just be held for a few minutes while you wait for his BG to rise, or perhaps you will have to encourage him to rest for a few minutes rather than returning to play.

With high blood sugars, your child will likely not notice feeling bad until his sugar is relatively high. Many parents first notice their child becoming thirsty and cranky when their sugar levels begin increasing. If he gets too high, it can potentially take several hours for the BG to return to normal once an insulin correction is given. During this time, your child may desire to go play, or again, he may just want to be held and loved.

Although your child is still young, let me encourage you to allow your child to take part in caring for himself. Don't pressure him, but he may ask to test himself, draw up insulin, or even inject himself. Of course you need to supervise, and even assist the really young ones, but it gives your youngster the opportunity to feel more in control of his circumstances. Don't be afraid to arrange to prick yourself a time or two to demonstrate (be sure to always use a clean lancet or needle, and do not use any solution in the syringe!). This also gives him the opportunity to want to imitate you, and the procedure becomes more like a game. There was a time when my two year old was "not quite right." For several days, I was instructed to prick his finger and test his blood periodically. When the nurse first told me that, I thought, "There is no way my toddler will let me do that more than once!" To my surprise however, he thought it was cool to be like mom. He had seen me test my blood sugar, and despite the sting of the lancet, you could tell he was fascinated by the blood appearing on his finger, the numbers counting down on the meter, and so forth. We made a game of it, and he never gave me a hassle throughout the ordeal. Now, several years later, he will periodically come to me when I am testing and say something like, "I need to check *my* blood; my sugar's low!" With a child this age, you can make the process easier by using fun, creative ideas that tailor to your child's interests and imagination.

If your child is wearing a pump, there are safeguards available to prevent the child from interfering with the settings. You can use safeguards on the pump itself, use a back harness system to keep the pump out of his reach, and even put his site into his back fat. Use the rule of thumb "out of sight, out of mind."

Grade Schooler

This age group absorbs information quickly, which can be a good thing and a bad thing. She can understand that she has a medical condition and needs special care. That can potentially make her more cooperative with testing and insulin regimens. A younger child may not be able to comprehend terms like "disease" without conjuring up images seen on television, while an older child may be perfectly comprehensive of the idea. In either case, she is at an age where you can begin training her to take care of herself. This will also take some of the responsibility off you. She could likely test herself and tend to certain parts of the insulin regimen, and she can be taught the difference between typical foods such as breads, meats, fruits, and vegetables. She can probably understand basic portion sizes. She should be recognizing some symptoms of a high or low blood sugar reaction. In addition to the other symptoms, like the younger children, she may be very hungry during a low. Help her learn to monitor what she eats, and only consume the amount of carbs necessary to stabilize her BG level. If she wants a snack, teach her to munch on protein or vegetables. At this age, she likely isn't yet embarrassed to have you around her friends, but realize that time may arrive before you know it. Start teaching her how to care for herself now so she is ready when you aren't there. If your child is older, you can begin to casually introduce the idea of complications, and help her begin to understand the reasons behind taking care of herself.

Between lessons on diet and dosing, your child will want to forget she is diabetic. She can now understand that she is "different" than her friends, and may begin to desire to hide her condition from others. She may be self-conscious and worried her friends will exclude her. Then again, she may be perfectly fine with it. However she is reacting to the situation, remember, nobody wants to hear the same thing over and over, and no diabetic wants to be continually reminded of their condition. So, as a parent, do what you have to do to ensure her health and safety, and then back off. Let her be a child. Be sure to treat her the same way you would treat a non-diabetic child. Let her "forget" sometimes that anything is wrong. Be aware that blood sugars may be difficult to control during growth spurts due to hormones, but this is normal. Don't overburden your child with the stress of perfection. If she is embarrassed or ashamed of her diabetes, then try not to talk about it with others when she is around. When possible, allow her to participate in your conversations with the doctor so she doesn't feel excluded. If you need to have a private conversation about her, then try to arrange a separate meeting or phone call when your child is absent and unaware.

At this age, she also wants to feel you will always be there if she needs you. Even when you aren't present physically, she needs to know that if she doesn't feel good, you have taught her, a school nurse, or other adult what to do to help her and how to find you. This information will help prevent her being afraid of being away from you for extended periods, which will help encourage her to live a normal life.

Tween-Teen

This age group brings a whole new set of issues. Your child will have a full understanding of diabetes, as well as the fact that he or she is somewhat different than peers. They may be self-conscious, embarrassed, or ashamed, or they may be totally carefree. You will find teenage hormones will drastically affect blood sugar levels and emotions. It is even more crucial that you discuss the dangers of drugs, alcohol, and unplanned pregnancy, emphasizing the added dangers of being a diabetic. Whether your teen has been recently diagnosed, or is a lifetime diabetic, throughout the teen years, they will most likely experience some physical and emotional issues specific to having diabetes. Also realize that you may loose a great deal of your control on your child at this point. If you push too hard for perfection in diabetes control, your teen may rebel somehow. Friends, however, may still have a great influence on your child. If they have drifted off to the "wrong" crowd of friends, there is a good chance it will only worsen the situation. Encouraging them to "hang with the good crowd" on the other hand, may help them through those tough years.

The one exception to the previous suggestion of not pushing for perfection is when your child is old enough to drive a vehicle. Require, in whatever way necessary, that your child test regularly before driving. If they are driving long distances, they should pull over and test every couple of hours and at any time they don't feel right. Modern meters have memories that will allow you to check if necessary to ensure your child is testing regularly before getting behind the wheel. This is not only necessary to protect them, but also to protect others.

When he reaches dating age, teen boys may be self-conscious about asking girls out. Like any parent, you can encourage social activities, but don't push too hard. Help your son understand the signals of a girl's interest. He may have no "girl troubles." Then again, he might. If he tends to be self-conscious about his diabetes, before he asks her out, let him know that if she says, "No," it is not necessarily because of his disease. If he is experiencing rejection, discuss with him how some girls can be very insensitive and rude, but that other girls know how to see past physical issues. He just has to find those girls, and the more involved he is, the easier it will be.

If you have a teen girl, buckle up! It will be a bumpy ride! Once she hits puberty and begins menstruating, your daughter's hormones will send her blood sugars all over the place. Documentation is the key to finding the patterns that she will exhibit with every cycle. Be patient as her body finds its unique cycle, as it may not happen right away. Ask your doctor how to adjust her insulin based on the requirements of individual days or weeks of the cycle. When she becomes interested in boys, she, too, will have fears of rejection. She may begin to question whether anyone will love her with her disease. She may question whether she can have babies and be a mother, and if so, what the chances are she will pass her diabetes on to her children. Just be there for her. Hear her out, and let her cry on your shoulder when necessary. Even if you notice a pattern of self-pity revolving around the monthly cycle or in relation to blood sugar levels (which is very possible), realize that she still has those feelings. At that moment, she needs a friend and confidant. Later, when she is feeling better, you can point out the trend if necessary, as well as suggest a plan to deal with those feelings.

When your teen is old enough to begin thinking about college or moving out, be sure you are supportive, despite how nervous you may be. If you could see past all the excitement, chances are you would see your teen is just as nervous. However, he or she has a desire to be independent. Whether they are looking forward to a career, following in friends' footsteps, or just wanting to start the next chapter of life, they need to know that you can appreciate that desire, and can support their decision. Focus your energies on helping them prepare for life as an independent adult, including emergency plans, diabetes care and maintenance, working with insurance companies, placing supply orders, and any other necessary topic. Your child will remember and appreciate your supportive efforts for the rest of their lives!

For Parents of Type 2 Children

If you are the parent of an overweight Type 2 diabetic child, it is imperative that changes be made. I realize I may step on some toes here, but the fact is, you are literally loving your child to death by allowing or even encouraging their current lifestyle. I never heard of a child with Type 2 when I was growing up. However, with obesity becoming more prevalent in our society, there are new children being diagnosed with Type 2 every day. It is an unfortunate fact. Because I grew up with Type 1 diabetes, never having the option of prevention or cure, my heart aches for young children who are suffering through daily meds or injections because of a disease that, in their case, was likely preventable. Fortunately, it may not be too late.

I implore you to heed your physician's advice, and make the changes necessary for your child's survival. Get them outside to play or exercise, and clean out the cupboards. This may sound a little crazy, but in order to ensure my children grow up active, we actually got rid of our television for a few years to help us break our bad television habits. Now that we have one again, we refuse to get cable or satellite, and limit the television to one or two videos a week. We don't own any video games, and we encourage our children to play outside whenever possible. You don't necessarily need to go that far, but you are the parent, and while your child lives in your house, your rules should apply. Set limits on television, computer, and video games. Monitor snacks and meals. Work with your child's doctor to develop a plan of action to get their weight under control. And, of course, you need to set the example. Despite what they may say to you now, they will likely thank you later.

Remember, your children are often a mirror image of you. I know from experience that weight loss, lifestyle changes, and sacrifice is difficult. However, it is imperative that you set the example for your child. Such changes will benefit your whole family, and could potentially save your child's life in the long run.

6

Just for Spouses of Diabetics

Perhaps you are considering marrying a diabetic, have recently married one, or your spouse has recently been diagnosed. Whichever is the case, you may be a little nervous about the responsibility you are accepting in this relationship, and you probably fear for your spouse's life. I expect you want to encourage your spouse to live as healthy as possible so they will survive as long as possible. The intent of this chapter is to offer tips and suggestions based on my experiences and conversations with my husband as we adapted to life as a married couple, as well as encounters and discussions with other couples affected by the disease.

Diabetes can certainly make a marriage relationship more interesting, to say the least. In addition to normal marital issues, diabetes brings high and low BG reactions to the mix. During a reaction, your diabetic spouse may be moody, emotional, introverted, or any combination therein. Please understand that this is a normal occurrence, and don't take it personally. A high blood sugar can leave your spouse feeling quite badly and low on energy. A low blood sugar can temporarily affect the way the brain functions. If your spouse experiences these highs or lows during the night, it can result in poor sleep and overall fatigue the following day. If roller-coaster BGs are a common occurrence, realize that all you can do is encourage your spouse to take control of their disease and get stable, then assist when necessary. If your spouse needs to find a new doctor, then help find one. Even if your insurance doesn't pay, many doctors will work with you on payment plans or even cash discounts. If your spouse is not willing to take the steps needed, understand that you cannot change a person who doesn't want to change. Frustrating as it may be for you, your hands are tied. There are, however, a few steps you can take to encourage this change, or even to support a spouse who is trying to maintain control.

First, if you are in charge of the grocery shopping, carefully consider the foods you choose to stock your pantry with. Try to limit high or simple carbohydrate foods, and eliminate sugary foods and drinks. Read nutrition labels, and purchase only those foods that encourage healthy eating habits. While they may resist at first, your spouse will likely appreciate your efforts— especially if they see you are sacrificing with them. If you bake, reduce the sugar content. I have found that most recipes will work out just fine with half, or even less, of the sugar called for in the recipe. This will significantly reduce carb and calorie intake. (please see Chapter 4 for more information).

A big issue unique to couples is the sexual part of the relationship. If your spouse uses an insulin pump, the two of you will have to learn to deal with inconvenient tubing and the pump itself. With the pump or injections, your spouse may eventually be faced with highs or lows, and untimely blood tests and snacks during an intimate moment. Shortly before, during, or after a high or low, a diabetic woman may experience a lack of lubrication or an inability to climax. I recommend keeping a tube of lubricating jelly handy for such moments. A diabetic man, particularly one who has had diabetes several years, has been in poor control, or is suffering a high or low blood sugar level, may experience impotence. In either case, it is crucial to your relationship that the non-diabetic spouse does not take the situation personally. It can be frustrating and embarrassing, but I can guarantee that the frustration you are feeling is mild in comparison with what your diabetic spouse is feeling. As the diabetic, your spouse likely feels betrayed by their body, and they may feel like a failure because of their seeming inability to control their body better. What your spouse needs more than anything during a moment like this is the assurance that you totally understand and still love them and their body. Your spouse's personality will determine how you show that understanding and love, but somehow, they need to know. Your relationship will be much better because of it.

Another area where you have every right to get involved is in regards to your spouse driving a vehicle. While you can't check their BG meter's memory without causing resentment, like parents can with their teens, you can certainly sit down and discuss what it means to you to know that they are as safe as they can be when driving. If your spouse is driving with children in the car, it is even more important. There are far too many stories of accidents and needless deaths due to a diabetic getting low, passing out, or having a seizure while driving. Such accidents are totally preventable most of the time. Anytime a diabetic is behind the wheel, they need to know what their blood sugar is doing. That may require hourly, or even more frequent, tests, or it may just mean a single test before heading out.

If children are in your future, you have additional things to consider first. Ideally, you will plan for the pregnancy, and a diabetic woman should work closely with doctors to stabilize BGs as necessary prior to getting pregnant. Pregnancies with Type 1 diabetes put a woman at high risk for several conditions, and the two of you should be educated. She may experience a perfectly normal, full-term pregnancy, or she could experience one or more complications. Every woman and every pregnancy is different. If she does experience complications, be careful to just support her. She will likely be questioning her decision to get pregnant, and blaming herself, or possibly even you, for anything that goes wrong. She needs your strength and understanding. Even if the pregnancy itself is normal, she may experience tremendous difficulty in maintaining tight BG control as her pregnancy progresses. Again, just be there for her and encourage her to do whatever she needs to do. Once the baby is born, she may battle low blood sugars for a time, especially if she chooses to nurse the baby. Whether mom or dad is diabetic, precautions need to be taken when the children are left alone with the diabetic parent. The two of you should develop a plan for extended time alone, such as checking in with someone routinely, and you should determine emergency plans. As the child matures, you can include them in your plans such as teaching them how to call 911 if mommy gets "sick and won't wake up."

I would also recommend you teach your spouse all the details regarding your diabetes care. As applicable, he or she should know how to dose medications, draw up insulin, give injections, administer Glucagon in an emergency, program an insulin pump, insert pump sites, and order and pick up supplies from the pharmacy. I learned from personal experience how beneficial this tip can be. At one point, I was in the hospital and due to complications from the delivery of my baby, passed out. Because of my husband's knowledge of the care I needed, the doctor actually allowed him to be in charge of my insulin and BG testing, rather than the nurses. He cared for me for several hours until I regained consciousness. See the "Medical Situations" section in Chapter 3.

Finally, don't continually harp on your spouse about diabetes-related issues. Although they have likely accepted their disease by now, there are still times when they will just want to forget they are diabetic for a moment and splurge somehow. Certainly talk to your spouse, find out what they want and need from you, and then drop it. Continually bringing up the same topics will likely result in resentment and possibly even rebellion against you or their diabetes.

7

Just For Diabetic Women

Women have unique hormonal issues that can potentially affect blood sugars drastically. This chapter is designed to help you prepare yourself to handle those factors. The key, as always, is to be very aware of, and in tune, to your body.

Monthly Cycle

Your monthly cycle and PMS-related factors are one of the more common causes of unexplained abnormal blood sugars. If you are unaffected by your monthly cyclic processes, you are a rare case. If you are not in tight control, you may not be aware of these changes. Chances are, you will experience changes dependant on the stage of your cycle you are entering. Whether your BG levels increase or decrease at each stage is something you will have to discover. To give you a clearer picture of what I am describing here, I will use the changes I experience throughout my cycle as an example.

About two days before my period actually starts, my sugars tend to increase drastically. As a result, I have to increase my basal rates by about three units in a 24 hour period. About 48 hours after it starts, my sugars decrease. I lower my basal rate by about five units per 24 hours. I become much more sensitive to insulin and activity, and can get low very easily. After my period stops, my BG levels gradually increase for a few days, then stabilize for about two weeks. Around the time of ovulation, my BGs take a big jump upward, and I become very resistant to insulin. I actually take several units more in a 24 hour period. This rate lasts about two weeks, until the increase in BGs signals that my period is about to begin. Throughout the entire cycle, my daily basal rates change from about 12 units at the lowest point to 20 units at the highest point.

I know of other women who are the exact opposite, with BGs increasing during their period and plummeting after ovulation. You will have to pay close attention to your body, your cycle, your BG levels, and your insulin rates for several cycles to find out how your body reacts. Keep good records during this time, and you will see a pattern. If you tend to have a regular cycle, it is much easier to predict, and therefore prevent, drastic BG level changes by changing your insulin rate just before you expect the BGs to change. If you have an irregular and unpredictable cycle, you can still do it, but you may have to wait until you have a day of unexplained BG levels to know it is time for the insulin change. In either case, if you happen to be on a pump, this could make the insulin changes much easier.

Some pumps actually offer methods of storing different insulin "patterns," allowing you to choose which pattern you want at that time. If your pump does not offer this option, just write down your basal rates before you change them. Compile a list of your differing rates, and keep the list handy so you know which rates you need to set at the appropriate time.

Pregnancy

For many years, women with diabetes were discouraged from becoming pregnant and having babies. With modern day advances, however, many diabetic women are doing just that. So what's the big deal?

Before even considering pregnancy, you need to get control of your lifestyle. The difficulty and frustrations of managing your BG levels without the pregnancy factor is nothing compared to what you will face while pregnant. In addition, just the fact that you are diabetic puts you and your unborn baby at high risk for several complications. Before you begin planning, I highly recommend you talk to your doctor and heed his advice. If he is unsure, ask for a consult with a perinatologist who regularly works with diabetics. Such a specialist can offer tremendous insight that will help you in your decision. Ultimately, however, the choice and responsibility is yours. That being said, if you are willing to go the distance, commit to the control that will be required during pregnancy, and work closely with your doctors, you may have a very good chance of having a healthy baby.

Before Getting Pregnant

You should allow yourself plenty of time to prepare your body for pregnancy. Pregnancy takes a toll on the body, and the body needs to be ready for the stress it will endure. Work with your doctor, and get your BG levels and HgbA1C's to a safe, healthy level. This is not as simple as it sounds.

Every doctor I saw before and during my pregnancies, to include two endocrinologists, a perinatologist, and an ophthalmologist, disagreed on what levels were ideal. One endocrinologist suggested BGs around 120 and an HgbA1C around 6, while the other recommended BGs between 80-100 and HgbA1C's around 5.5. The perinatologist preferred BGs around 70 and HgbA1C's around 5, as the babies seem to have less difficulty after birth. The ophthalmologist wanted BGs around 140 and

HgbA1C's around 6.5 to prevent eye problems often developed during pregnancy. Your first step is to find good doctors to walk you through your pregnancy. Similar to your search for a good endocrinologist or diabetes specialist, ask questions. Find out what the doctor's background and experience is, and what they have in mind for your appointments. What is the plan for delivering a best-case scenario and worst-case scenario? Will the pregnancy specialist allow you to work with the endocrinologist as well, or will that cause issues and confusion? As you can see, there are many opinions, and there may even be legitimate reasons, however, once again, the choice is ultimately yours. I chose to stick with the "normal" non-diabetic BG range of 80-100, and HgbA1C's between 5.2 and 5.8. My doctors agreed to work with me as a team, where all pregnancy-related questions and situations were handled by my perinatologist, and all diabetes-related issues were handled by my endocrinologist. If I had an issue that fell somewhere in between, then I would often discuss it with both doctors, and decide from there. Find what works for you and your baby.

Once you get your BGs and HgbA1C's to your target levels, try to keep them there for several months prior to getting pregnant. This will help you develop some habits you will need during pregnancy, as well as help you tune in closely to your body. It is also a good idea to have a complete physical done during this time. Have your eyes checked for any sign of damage, as well as a urine test to check for kidney damage. Your doctor should also run a full panel of blood work. Also, pay a visit to the dentist. Be aware that if signs of complications are found during the tests, your doctor may discourage you from getting pregnant, either temporarily or permanently. To an extent, many complications may be reversed, or at least prevented from progressing by tightening control of your diabetes. If you are able to reverse damage, you may still be able to carry to term safely.

During Pregnancy

Just as pregnancy affects every woman differently, it affects every diabetic differently. Once you are pregnant, it is more crucial than ever to tighten and maintain good BG control. If you happen to discover you are pregnant, and did not have a chance to plan, just make changes as needed. It's always better late than never. Fortunately, women have a two-week "grace period" between conception and the development of the placenta and umbilical cord. Circumstances are more critical in regards to the baby after that grace period has ended and the umbilical cord begins functioning.

You have likely heard all the typical horror stories of pregnancy, and many of them were probably related to diabetic pregnancies. First and foremost, realize that women have been having babies for thousands of years. While a few result in some type of difficulty or complication, the great majority result in healthy babies. Diabetes certainly adds increased levels of difficulty and risk, but the levels can be significantly reduced by maintaining good blood sugar control.

The First Trimester

While every woman's body is affected differently, generally speaking, the first trimester is typically the second most challenging time for a diabetic mother-to-be. As pregnancy hormones within the body begin raging, many women, whether or not they are diabetic, experience symptoms such as nausea, fatigue, intense hunger (or a total loss of appetite). In addition to normal pregnancy symptoms, diabetics often experience a drastic decrease in their BG levels due to the hormone changes and the increased workload of nourishing a developing baby. As a result, you need to work with your doctor to lower your insulin levels as needed. I was fortunate to not have to deal with daily morning sickness; however, I have had diabetic friends who did. If you are one of the latter, you must take extra care not to inadvertently overdose with insulin, if there will not be food left to counteract that insulin. I recommend keeping juice boxes handy for the duration of this trimester. I was, however, cursed with major, intense hunger sensations that would hit fast and hard. If I didn't eat within ten minutes, I would vomit. One of my favorite solutions for this problem was a drink designed for diabetics called "Glucerna." Similar to a diet shake, it would quickly soothe my stomach, while providing some extra energy and nutrition. In addition, it was balanced with proteins and fiber to help stabilize blood sugar.

If the baby is going to develop physical complications or deformities, it will generally happen during the first trimester. While consistently low blood sugars can cause problems with the baby, they are often related more to the brain function. Consistently high blood sugars can result in physical deformity. While controlling BG levels doesn't guarantee a healthy baby, it certainly guarantees a better chance of one.

Just like in routine diabetes management, every doctor has personal opinions and preferences as to the pre-natal care you should receive. Like my specialist during my second pregnancy, yours may want to see you on a weekly basis, and even perform an ultrasound several times per month. Or, like my diabetic friends' doctors, yours may only want to see you every three months, and perform only two ultrasounds the entire pregnancy. The frequency is not really that crucial, assuming you are generally a healthy diabetic, in good control. The worse your BG control, the more frequently you should be in contact with a specialist in order to prevent problems. More important is your understanding of what to do should different situations arise. You will likely have some questions and concerns throughout the course of your pregnancy. Your doctor should be willing to answer those questions and help you develop a game plan. However, realize that your doctor is likely a very busy person who hears the same questions several times each day. Try not to take it personally if he doesn't seem as concerned as you feel. I found through my pregnancies, my questions were more likely to get answered if they were actually written on a list. When the doctor walked in and asked how I was feeling, I would inform him up front that I had several questions. Then, depending on how busy he was, we would discuss the questions either during or after my exam. Another tip is to organize your questions based on importance to you. There may be times where your doctor will be unable to answer an entire list, so if you can at least ask the ones that are most important, you will feel much more at ease with asking the remaining questions at the following visit. As an additional note, don't hesitate to talk to the doctor's nurse. The nurse usually has a little more time, and often has the knowledge to answer common questions.

The Second Trimester

You have probably heard that the second trimester is the easiest for women as a whole, and the same applies for diabetics. During the second trimester, the baby has formed, and then begins to simply grow. Organs also begin to develop and function on their own to some extent. You will likely not be as tired, and you may notice a slight increase in your BG levels. While you may have to increase your insulin levels for a while, as a general rule, the levels will stabilize within a couple of weeks. You will get a break for a while from the constant worry about lows and unpredictable BGs. I found the second trimester to be the easiest time of my life when it came to controlling BG levels. Since I was pregnant, I didn't have the monthly cycle of hormones changing my BG patterns every week or so. Rather, once they stabilized, my insulin patterns remained at the same level for about two and a half months.

If you have been diabetic for many years, you may notice a lot of round-ligament pains. This baffled me for a while until a doctor explained that long-term diabetics seem to have less elasticity of the tissues. I actually began experiencing crippling pains during the first trimester. Once, I was hit so badly with pain that I was left in the fetal-position, unable to lie flat for about 12 hours. My doctor recommended a decrease in activity, which helped tremendously. This will not necessarily be the case in your pregnancy, but I thought it was worth mentioning in the event your doctor cannot explain it. Along these same lines, you may notice early development of stretch marks. The less elastic your skin, the earlier your stretch marks will develop and more prevalent they may be.

A potential plus of being diabetic is that you may feel fetal movement earlier than many women. This does, of course, vary with each woman, and other factors such as your weight and the placenta and baby's position will also be contributing factors. However, because you may be more in tune with your body, you may notice little flutters earlier than the average woman. I am generally considered to have a "fit" body style, and am very tuned in. As a result, I felt my first sure kick during an ultrasound when I was only 13 weeks pregnant with my first, and 15 weeks with my second. Learning your body certainly has its advantages!

Around week 16, your baby's pancreas will begin producing its own insulin. At that point, you can relax even more, because he will no longer be affected as greatly by your high blood sugar levels. However, you will still want to be cautious about having too many highs, as your baby will begin to store the excess glucose as fat. An overly fat baby can have complications during and after the delivery. If he has become used to the high glucose levels, the baby may also experience very low blood sugars for a while after delivery, once the umbilical cord is cut..

The Third Trimester

If you haven't already, now is the time to begin educating yourself on potential complications of a diabetic pregnancy. If you have worked closely with your doctor, you likely have a good idea regarding the baby's health and development. During the third trimester, the baby continues to grow. In the latter half, the baby begins to gain fat to help him in the world he is about to enter.

There are many resources where you can find out more information about diabetes-related complications and risk, so I will not go into detail here. However, a few worth mentioning are high-blood pressure, pre-eclampsia, toxemia, pre-term labor, early placental deterioration, and premature delivery. Despite how your pregnancy may go, the baby may experience complications such as being very large, under-developed lungs, low blood sugars, and jaundice. Keep in mind, these are complications that could potentially affect any woman or baby, but diabetics are at a slightly higher risk. Several are directly related to blood sugar levels. Once again, the more controlled your BGs, the less the risk to you and your baby.

One difficulty you will almost certainly encounter as you progress through your third trimester is an increase in your insulin resistance. You will likely notice drastic, unexplainable increases in your BG levels, which can only be treated with large increases in your insulin levels. To give you an example, in my second pregnancy, I went from about 18 total units per day in my early second trimester, to about 100 units per day by the time of delivery. There are always exceptions, but you should be prepared for this to occur to some degree. In relation, you will likely notice a new level of sensitivity to foods. You may have to temporarily give up certain foods, or change the way you administer your insulin. For example, about half way through the third trimester in both my pregnancies, I learned that my body could not handle carbs such as pasta and rice, and it couldn't handle more than about 20 carbs at any given time. If I ate more than that amount, my BG level would shoot to 400 within an hour, and it would take about 15 units and four hours to come down. By working closely with my doctors, we developed a plan that helped tremendously. If my sugar was over 160, I ate nothing or limited a meal to protein and vegetables. If I was between 100 and 160, I could eat about 15 carbs, if I took my insulin 20 minutes prior to eating and ate protein first. Below 100, I was allowed to eat 20 carbs and bolus 10 minutes prior. And if I was below 70, I could bolus when I ate and add a single serving of fruit to my meal. As difficult as this may sound, it is doable. Although the reactions may change somewhat, it is much easier if you have already familiarized yourself with your body's "normal" reactions to foods prior to this point.

Pregnancy can be an emotional roller-coaster without diabetes, but when you factor in diabetes, don't be surprised if you experience moments of intense stress. I can speak from experience about how frustrating it can be to work as hard as possible to maintain tight control, give up everything you like to eat, and still have things go wrong. In addition to insulin resistance, I experienced several complications—some diabetes-related, most not related. I was blessed with a wonderful husband and nurse who let me cry on their shoulders in moments of intense frustration, and two doctors who just sat and listened to my concerns and offered sincere empathy for my situation. Between the four of them, I was given some wonderful advice. To paraphrase, "You can only do your best, and then you must trust God, nature, and the doctor to take care of things. Stressing out will not help the situation, and in fact, may make it worse. So do what you can, and then try to enjoy the remaining few weeks of the miracle of pregnancy."

During and After Birth

Like the majority of women, you may be blessed to have a perfectly normal delivery. There are a few things to be aware of, however. It is very normal for your baby to experience a few low blood sugars shortly after delivery. If you happen to hear the BG number, don't panic. Newborns may experience BGs as low as 30, but 50 is more common. According to my doctors, these lows do not affect a newborn the same way as an older infant, child, or adult. In order to treat the low, however, be aware that the doctor may choose to send the baby to the NICU for monitoring and give the baby some formula or glucose water. In more severe cases, the baby may need an I.V. of dextrose solution to help his sugars stabilize. If you prefer to nurse, feel free to ask the doctor if you can nurse to treat the low. If he thinks additional treatment is needed, however, don't fret, as this treatment will likely be temporary and it will not prevent the baby from nursing later.

Jaundice is another common problem with newborns, but particularly with babies of diabetic mothers. If this is the case with your baby, talk to the doctor about feeding preferences, lights, and home treatments. Depending on the severity, your doctor may be very flexible in treatment, or he may want to put the baby on a formula regimen and keep him under lights 24 hours a day for several days. In either case, again, keep in mind that there are options in any circumstance, if you have educated yourself. Most doctors would allow a mother to nurse between or before bottles or even pump bottles. If you aren't interested in nursing, then you may enjoy sharing responsibilities of feeding the baby with others so you can have a break. My three older children all dealt with jaundice to different degrees. My first son required bili lights in the hospital for three days, and was sent home with a bili blanket he was required to use for the next two weeks. My daughter required just 24 hours of lights in the hospital, while my second son (whose birthmother had gestational diabetes) showed some yellowing of the eyes, but never required lights. Whatever happens, just keep in mind that jaundice is usually a temporary and very treatable condition.

If you plan to nurse, but one or both of these situations arise and your baby's doctor recommends formula supplementation, don't lose hope. My first baby had low blood sugars for about three hours after birth, and required supplemental formula during that time. He later developed severe jaundice, and due to my low milk production, he was supplemented with formula almost every two hours for two weeks. When my milk finally increased, he went on to nurse successfully for over eight months. My second baby experienced very low blood sugars for almost four hours after birth, requiring monitoring in the NICU during that time. She later developed a mild case of jaundice. She, too, was given supplemental formula, but went on to nurse successfully.

Your body will also go through many changes in a very short period of time. It is likely you will need a decrease in insulin during labor, and once you birth the placenta, you may need very little to no insulin for several hours, or even a couple of days after the birth. If you decide to nurse, you may notice a pattern of low BG levels around the time of nursing. My dietician at the time recommended that I drink a glass of milk every time I sat down to nurse, and that I keep a juice box handy just in case. This tip helped me tremendously. Again, all the above changes are due to the many physiological changes that take place during this time. You may be affected by them little or greatly. I just want you to be aware so you can discuss a plan with your doctor in advance.

8

So You're Considering a Pump?

There are several methods of administering insulin, including, but not limited to, syringes, high-pressured injector pens, and infusion pumps. All have their advantages and disadvantages, and you must decide what works best for you. If you are considering a new method, I encourage you to talk to your doctor and research, research, research. Talk to anyone you encounter who uses other methods and find out why they do, or do not, like the method. Because there seem to be many misguided beliefs about the pump, I am going to focus on the increasingly popular insulin pump in this chapter. Although I prefer a pump over any other option available today, I do *not* believe it is right for everyone, and I will explain why throughout this chapter.

Insulin pumps were basically developed to help make artificial insulin delivery as natural as possible. Remember, in a healthy body, the pancreas releases small basal doses of insulin throughout the day, and quick boluses of insulin to cover food or other factors affecting BG levels. When a person is on injections, they typically take long-acting insulin once or twice per day that acts as a basal. Occasionally, they will then take a fast-acting bolus injection at meal times. However, using this method, there tends to be a "peak" of insulin, followed shortly by a rapid decrease in levels available. These peaks tend to cause lows. Since the low must be treated with carbs, and the peak is followed by a decrease in insulin levels, then there is often a high BG level shortly thereafter. There are many people who successfully maintain their BG target levels using injections, however, for those who don't know how, or perhaps just desire more flexibility, rigid control can be difficult. So, the pump is the next best thing available to a real pancreas.

The pump is a pager-sized computer that holds a reservoir of insulin which is connected to a tube. The tube then carries the insulin into the body through a small cannula or needle. The pump computer stores programmed information. Like the pancreas, it then uses this information to release small, pre-set basal doses of insulin throughout the day. When you eat, you program a bolus into the computer, which is administered as programmed. If your BG level gets high, you can also program a "correction bolus" of insulin to be administered immediately to help bring the level back to target range.

Advantages

A pump has many wonderful and beneficial advantages. Depending on the type of pump used, it may have the ability to store different basal patterns for use on different days. They have special security systems and safety checks to ensure all computer and delivery systems are functioning as desired. Some offer the ability to choose basal rates in hundredth unit increments, while others are whole unit increments. Some offer the option of setting multiple bolus rates, or "ratios," at different times of the day, and work with your BG monitor to document BG levels and recommend correction doses. Several have software programs that allow you to download information onto your computer, making record-keeping easier, and some are even designed to work with new glucose monitoring systems.

Outside of physical characteristics, the pump is well known for the increased BG control, freedom, and convenience it allows users. Tight control has been known to stop progression of complications, or even reverse it in some cases. There is often a choice of "sites," or the part that actually goes into your skin, so you can choose which works best with your skin. Because only fast-acting insulin is used, and the way the insulin is administered, the pump allows more flexibility at meal times, during illness or exercises, and during vacations and travel. This flexibility can be used to help prevent low or high BG levels.

Disadvantages

The pump also has its share of disadvantages you should carefully consider. While the pump's size is usually small and discreet, you are attached to it 24 hours a day. Though some versions can be disconnected along the tubing or site temporarily, it is usually recommended you wear it at all times. This includes while swimming, showering, sleeping, working, playing sports, etc. Because the insulin is fast-acting, if there happens to be a problem with the site or tubing, or you run out of insulin, your BG level can increase rapidly. Likewise, if you take a bolus, your BG can drop rapidly. It generally takes about four to five hours for a dose of insulin to be completely used up in your body. As a result, if you turn the pump off, you may still have low BG values due to the residual insulin in your system. Whereas injections allow fresh insulin to be inserted into fresh tissue each time, the pump site administers insulin into the same tissue until it is changed. Additionally, because the reservoir of insulin is located inside the pump, and the pump is typically worn close to the body, the insulin warms over time. These latter two factors can result in poor insulin quality over the several days it remains in the reservoir, as well as some resistance and problems with the tissue around the site. For these reasons, it is recommended that you change your site every three days (or less), and that you test regularly—sometimes more frequently than when using other methods of insulin delivery. I go a step further when I need to treat a high BG level with more than one unit of insulin, and give myself an injection of fresh insulin. By not using the pump for that treatment, I prevent added stress to the surrounding tissues, and my BG level seems to return to normal range significantly faster. Also, because the site contains an adhesive and must be stuck to your skin, you can potentially get rashes, itchiness, or other reactions to the site. If you are a traveler, or must otherwise frequently pass through metal detecting machines, the pump may potentially cause delays. While many pumps can safely pass through the machines, some may trigger the alarm, requiring you to be personally searched. Finally, a big disadvantage to the pump is the simple fact that it is your lifeline. Should the pump malfunction or suddenly stop working, you must have a backup plan.

As a side note, in the event of a pump failure, my doctor instructed me to write down my total *basal* amount of insulin for a 24 hour period. Should the pump fail, a long-acting insulin can be purchased without a prescription at any pharmacy. Divide the total basal in half, and, using regular insulin syringes, administer half before breakfast, and the other half before bed—with the injections about 12 hours apart. For example, if the total basal for the day is 24 units, you would inject 12 units at 7 a.m. and 12 units at 7 p.m. Then, give additional injections of the normal, short-acting insulin used in the pump before each meal or to treat a high BG level, using the same units-to-carbs ratio as used with the pump. This plan should be discussed with your doctor.

Selection

The process of selecting a pump can be quite overwhelming, as there are several brands and styles to choose from. I encourage you to research carefully. Some offer excellent customer support, while others do not. Because a pump is nothing more than a computer, it can have malfunctions. I recommend only considering a pump company that has 24 hour technical support available, a lengthy warranty (several years is preferable), as well as a program to supply you with a loaner or replacement pump while yours is repaired if necessary. These types of companies generally make excellent, reliable pumps that rarely have a problem, but when they do, the support is comforting. Ask for any free information available, talk to your doctor about what kind he recommends for you, and talk to other pump users about their experiences. I said ask your doctor for a recommendation, however, use caution with his answer. In many cases, the doctor has not thoroughly researched the different types of pumps available, and instead, has relied on the information provided by one or two sales people. Many doctors are also obligated by contract to recommend the style of pump sold by their contracted supplier, who often works in the doctor's office as a pump and/or diabetes educator. I have also had one doctor who refused to work with my pump company because he said they required him to do too much paperwork. So he limited his recommendation to a pump company who has a long history of pump problems. Just use your best judgment.

Realize that a pump cannot work miracles in your lifestyle. In fact, if you are not good with self-discipline, it can make living a healthy lifestyle more difficult, due to the freedom it allows. For this reason, a pump is not recommended for everyone. I know people who have been refused a pump because of their lifestyle, and others who have been given a pump, just to have it taken away because they lost control in their new-found freedom. The pump, no doubt, requires a balancing act of freedom and responsibility. You must be able to hold yourself accountable for things like eating correctly, counting carbohydrates, testing more frequently, etc. You must also be sure to order supplies on a regular basis. Pump supplies cannot be purchased from most pharmacies like syringes can, but usually must be ordered directly from a supplier. Therefore, you never want to be caught without refills and replacements. If you are unsure about the responsibility involved, or don't have the desire to do whatever it takes to stay healthy, the pump might not be for you. Along the same lines, if you have a child who is abusing the freedom allowed by the pump, talk to your doctor about removing the pump from your child's insulin regimen. While the pump helps prevent long-term complications, abuse of the pump can tremendously increase the risk of a severe or even fatal high or low BG level.

If, however, you think you are dedicated enough to your health to do whatever is required, than you may be a candidate. Consider what you might need from a pump. If you need the option of easily disconnecting from the pump on a regular basis, then you may want to stay with injections, or at least choose a pump that allows disconnecting as close to the skin as possible. If you require small amounts of insulin, you may need a pump that offers doses in partial-unit increments. If you are planning to get pregnant, or are very insulin resistant, then you may need a pump with a larger insulin reservoir. If you are considering the pump for a child, then you may want to consider one that is extra rugged and durable, and/or with the option of a "harness" or child-lock to prevent your child from tampering with the buttons. If you are a woman who wears one-piece dresses frequently, then you may want a pump that offers discreetness for wearing under the dress, such as hooked in your bra or on a band around your thigh. If you would like a "trial run" before committing, then consider wearing a pager or cell phone attached to you 24 hours per day, for a week or so. You could also ask your doctor if he has a loaner or demo pump that you could borrow for a week or so. In addition, begin testing your BGs a minimum of six times a day, if you don't already. You may have to increase your prescription allowance for test strips to do this. Discuss your considerations with your doctor, and decide what to do from there.

Just for the record, I have used a Medtronic Minimed pump for roughly 15 years. While I have had discussions with other pump users regarding different brands, I have no personal experience with other brands. However, I can say I have been very happy with Minimed, and I have found the following useful.

- Upgrade program--I have used three different versions of Minimed pumps over the years, upgrading to newer models when my warranties ran out.
- 24/7 Customer support--While I have had very few problems with the pump, when I have had an issue arise, the Minimed customer service has

been exceptional. They are on call for emergencies 24 hours a day, seven days a week.

- Loaner pump program--On one occasion, I did have a problem where my pump completely stopped working, and after a quick phone call to the support line, they sent out a loaner pump which arrived the very next morning.

- Support phone numbers printed on pump—I have had pump related questions many times when I was away from home, and it was wonderful to have the needed phone numbers and pump model info printed right on the back of the pump.

- Recessed reservoir tip—I used to use a pump in which the tip of the reservoir stuck out from the pump itself. As a result, I inadvertently bumped, snagged, and sliced open the tubing several times. More recent models have the reservoirs completely enclosed inside the pump, preventing this problem from occurring.

- $1/100^{th}$ unit increments—My current pump, a 508 model, will allow me to set my basal rates in $1/100^{th}$ unit increments. This factor has been a critical part of my success in BG control. Over the course of a day, $1/100^{th}$ of a unit adds up. When you factor in boluses for meals, snacks, and elevated BG levels, it may be several units a day difference.

- Meter to pump link feature—My current pump has a feature that uses infrared communication, allowing the meter to transmit BG data to the pump. This feature is useful with the Bolus Wizard, described next.

- Bolus Wizard Calculator—My current pump has a feature called "Bolus Wizard." This feature allows me to program my ratio of units insulin to carbs eaten. For example, I may need one unit of insulin for every 10 carbs I consume. After programming, I simply enter the number of carbohydrates I plan to eat, and the calculator will use BG data transmitted from the meter and the carb data I enter to recommend a precise amount of insulin for me to administer. If I approve the amount, I simply activate the bolus and that amount is administered.

- Delayed boluses—Several pumps have a feature such as the "Square Wave Bolus" or "Dual Wave Bolus," with which a bolus can be spread out over a set period of time. For example, if I overeat, as discussed in the "Food" section of Chapter 3, or eat a fatty meal such as pizza, a regular bolus will cause me to have a low BG shortly after the meal, followed by a rebounding high BG level. To prevent this, I can use the delayed bolus features to spread all or part of the bolus out over several hours.

- Auto Off Feature—This feature allows you to program the pump to turn off all insulin delivery if you don't press a button within a set amount of time. If it reaches that set time and turns off, it will sound an increasingly loud alarm. I used this feature frequently when I rode horses on the trail by myself. Because the horse-riding activity could potentially cause me to get low, I would program the pump to shut off after two hours. In the event I was thrown from the horse and knocked unconscious, this feature could potentially help in two ways. First, a bad situation could be made worse if the activity of riding caused a drop in BG, yet I continued getting insulin. If my BG level got high from the lack of insulin, on the other hand, the danger was not quite as great. Secondly, since I always told someone where I was going and when to expect me back, if I didn't return shortly after the given time, they would come search for me. The alarming pump could potentially help them find me sooner. Of course, this is just one example of how the feature could be used.

- Site disconnection—I find it absolutely necessary to be able to disconnect from my pump periodically. When my BG levels are stable, I prefer to disconnect to shower, swim, or during intimate moments with my husband. By being able to disconnect at the insertion site, I do not have to worry about extra tubing getting in the way of my activity.

- Computer downloads—I love being able to download all the data from my meter and my pump to my computer, and view the data using computerized logs, charts, and graphs. It makes diabetes maintenance between doctor visits much easier.

- Lock keypad feature—If I were to use this pump on a young child, this feature would be a requirement. It allows to you to lock the keypad, much like you would lock the keypad of a cell phone. This prevents the child from messing up any programmed settings or accidentally administering a bolus of insulin.

- Self Checks and Alarms—I find great comfort in the number of automatic safety checks performed by my pump, as well as the numerous alarms it will sound in the event a problem is discovered.

9

So You're Considering Continuous Glucose Monitoring?

There is a relatively new technology to help monitor and control blood sugars. It is known as continuous glucose monitoring. Only a few are currently approved for public use by the FDA.

The principle behind the CGM systems is to fill in the gaps left by routine blood testing, allowing more accurate development of blood glucose patterns, as well as to remove some of the guesswork from setting basals and administering boluses of insulin. The system generally consists of an electrode or wire-like device that is inserted into the skin. This device slightly resembles the site used by the insulin pump. Minimed's version is a thin Teflon cannula that contains the sensor measuring device inside. A monitor, or transmitter, is then attached to this sensor device. The monitors are pre-programmed to read glucose values every five to seven minutes, depending on the variety used. Some versions are designed for patients using injections rather than pumps, other brands are designed to work with your pump, which collects and stores all the information. The device is then programmed to read your glucose levels, and as levels reach pre-determined values, an alarm is set off to notify you. It has the potential to warn not only of a high or low value, but also to warn *prior* to the high or low, when it detects a rapid change in BG level. This allows you time to treat or prepare as necessary to prevent a more critical or dangerous problem later. Obviously, such early warnings and safety alarm systems can be a tremendous advantage over current standard testing methods.

Like all technology, the CGM systems have their disadvantages. Like the pump, it is a device that must be attached to your body in order to function as designed. This is an important factor. I have young children, and often have a baby sitting on my hip, therefore I have to make a conscious effort to position the sensor and my pump site in locations where they won't be inadvertently ripped out by my children. The adhesive and sensor could potentially cause skin reactions similar to pump sites. Due to the metal sensor device inside the cannula, the cannula itself, as well as the needle used to insert the cannula, is quite a bit larger in diameter than a traditional insulin syringe needle or pump site, potentially causing some discomfort upon insertion. When used correctly, if you have a bad night with lots of lows or highs, then you may get little sleep due to the alarms sounding. In addition, you do still have to test with a traditional meter in order to calibrate the system, but tests are decreased to about two times per day. The system should not be abused, and in fact, it is often recommended that a high or low reading be double checked with a standard finger-test reading before treating. One big reason is that the sensor measures your glucose reading in your cell's interstitial fluid, or the fluid that "bathes" your cells, rather than blood. Therefore, the glucose reading may differ, and actually lag about 15 minutes behind a blood glucose reading. So, your sensor may read you are 100, when in actuality you are 70 if your sugar levels tend to drop rapidly. On the other hand, your sensor may read 60, tempting you to treat a low, but if you test, your blood glucose reading may be 100. Also, you must change the sensor every three to seven days, depending on the brand used.

A CGM system is an option certainly worth considering and researching. If you and your doctor are able to see what your glucose values are doing throughout the day for multiple days, you can more accurately predict trends, estimate insulin levels, set carbohydrate rates, and prepare for problems. You learn how often you may "micromanage" your BG levels, meaning how often you tend to treat a perceived high or low blood sugar when you shouldn't have. For example, if you test with a meter and your BG level reads 180, you may be tempted to take a dose of insulin. With the CGM, however, you can see that your BG actually rose to 250, had already dropped back to 180, and was still dropping. So, in actuality, taking a dose of insulin would cause you to get low. As a result, with the CGM, you significantly reduce the chance of a severe high or low. This knowledge may also help you discover reasons for "unexplained" BG values. Be sure to get your doctor's recommendations and opinions before deciding, and, like the pump, be sure to ask questions to determine his or her reasoning. See the chapter "So You're Considering a Pump?" for some information and guidelines that may help you in your decision.

10

So You're Considering A Service Dog?

I mentioned in the "My Story" section of Chapter 1 that I used a Medical Alert Service Dog. I know from experience how difficult it can be to find more information about service dogs trained for diabetics, therefore I decided to include a brief chapter on the topic. If you think you may be interested in acquiring a Medical Alert Dog, I can offer some things you should consider first.

Owning and using a specially trained service dog is a true pleasure. The dogs are capable of amazing tasks from alerting and responding to low and high blood sugars, retrieving treatments such as juice, calling for help, stabilizing the owner during a weak or dizzy spell, and more. As amazing as they are, however, a service dog is still just a dog, despite the amount of training he or she has had. A dog is not a substitute for good diabetes management, regular testing, and conscious health choices. Rather, the dog is an additional option to assist with that management. Along with the many benefits the dog can offer, there are also many disadvantages and challenges. One very important note is that the dogs are generally trained specifically for compliant, insulin-dependent, diabetics. The level of compliancy required, however, is left to the training organization's discretion. The following is a list of questions you should ask yourself prior to considering a dog:

- Why do you think a service dog would be right for you?
- Can you handle keeping your dog with you *at all times*? This includes work, bed, car, school, church, restaurants, grocery shopping, restroom breaks, vacations, formal events, etc.
- Can you handle the frequent unwanted attention and direct questions regarding your dog and disability?
- Can you handle dog hair on every outfit, in your car, around your bed, and basically *everywhere*?
- Do you have the time necessary to devote to proper training reviews, hygiene care, and exercise for the dog?
- Can you afford high-quality veterinary care and food, which is vital to sustain your dog's regular and working life?
- Will your family, friends, and co-workers (or child's teachers, classmates, and their parents) support the idea of you having a dog with you?
- Can you discipline yourself to *NOT* feed the dog people food, table scraps, etc?
- Can you accept whatever breed of dog you receive, even if it isn't your "favorite" breed, color, or size? Likewise, can you accept a dog that is already named? Fact is you may not get any choice, other than whether or not you will accept a dog that the organization feels is a good match.
- Do you mind packing a "doggy bag" every time you leave home? Having a service dog can be a lot like having a toddler. They require certain supplies that you generally have to keep with you

or at least keep in your car where they are handy if you need them.

- If the dog is for a child, can the child handle the responsibility of a dog, both physically and emotionally?
- Are you able to take time off work and perhaps travel for initial training, any required certifications, bonding time, and possible follow ups?
- Finally, can you afford the cost of a service dog? It is a widely-known fact that the average finished service dog is worth about $25,000 to $40,000. While there is at least one training organization that has a donation and sponsor program allowing them to provide dogs to qualified diabetics for no charge, such a school may have a very lengthy waiting list (years long). Other organizations must charge to ensure their costs are covered, but on occasion they offer discounts or scholarship programs to help cover the cost. Even these organizations, however, may have lengthy wait times.

There is far too much information to list here when it comes to deciding whether a service dog is right for you. If you are still interested after answering the above questions, then I would encourage you to do some research on your own. Talk to someone who uses a service dog for more information regarding what daily life is like. While the dog may get to act like a pet during down-time, they are not a pet. They have rules that must be followed at all times. They are more of a lifestyle that requires a huge commitment and sometimes a great deal of effort. These dogs are either bred or chosen for their desire to work, therefore they thrive on the training they receive and love to perform their job. You must be at least as committed to them as they are to you for the relationship to work.

Should you decide to pursue getting an alert dog, let me warn you that there are many scam artists out there posing as qualified trainers. There are even so-called "organizations" and "training schools" that are good for little more than taking your hard-earned money. Use caution, and do your research on an organization before you decide to call them. Investigate their rating with the Better Business Bureau, and search the trainer or organization name on the internet and read the articles that may pop up. Finally, call them and ask questions. A reputable and proven trainer should be able and willing to answer your questions thoroughly. While most will not reveal the training techniques (understandably), they will offer guarantees, refunds, re-matches, follow-up services, etc. When I say guarantee, however, I am referring to a guarantee that they will match you with a dog that alerts, even if it takes several tries. Stay clear of anyone who guarantees that a particular dog will alert for you. Dogs have been known to alert for one person and not another, or alert during training but lose interest afterward. There are many factors that contribute to dog's success at alerting. Be as serious about this subject as you are about your disease. Research, ask questions, and educate yourself. Don't let yourself get into such a rush or get so excited or emotional that you neglect to listen to your gut instinct. Owning a dog as well-trained as these is a true blessing in many ways, but you must do your part if you want the experience to be a pleasant one.

As I mentioned in Chapter 1, I used to use a Medical Alert Service Dog, but had to retire him. It is worth

114

noting the reasons behind that retirement. You see, my dog was well trained, wonderful at alerting, and took his job very seriously. Even despite some very minor arthritis that had developed in one of his shoulders, he loved to work. However, after I had two children, it became much more difficult to be as attentive to him when he was working. Not only would I have to be aware of how my dog was behaving, but I also had to always be aware of my two young children. On two occasions this lack of attention came to a climax when, after arriving home from running errands, I got out of the car, took the kids out of their carseats, gathered the diaper bags, and miscellaneous items collected throughout our errands, and took everyone inside. Because my dog was so well-trained, he had a tendency to just wait patiently until I opened the back and let him out of the car. On these two occasions, however, his quiet behavior and my distractions resulted in him being forgotten and left in the car. I was very fortunate that I didn't loose him to overheating. I realized, though, that for his own safety, it was no longer wise to take him out with me. Because of his arthritis, and the fact that I was also using a Continuous Glucose Monitor, the decision was made easier to just allow him to live out the remainder of his life as a pet. I say the above to point out that, if you are interested in a service dog, you must consider all aspects of your life, and realize that the dog will add some degree of challenge to your current lifestyle.

11

Just Do It!

So you've done your research, you're working closely with a doctor, and you have a good understanding of how different factors affect your blood sugar levels. You may still be overwhelmed and confused. There will come a time when you have to just take things one day at a time. You may feel like diabetes care is the focus of your every waking minute. You may even dream about it at night. This is normal. Like anything, however, rest assured that it will eventually become second nature for you. You will learn how to count your carbs and dose your insulin as fast as you can answer the question, "What's your name?" If you take the time and make the effort now to learn about your body, everything will come easier later. Testing BG levels will become like a security blanket of sorts, where you just automatically want to test when you don't feel right, as compared to having to remember to test regularly.

It is important, however, not to stress or pressure yourself too much. High and low BGs are expected once in a while. Particularly if you are on insulin, you cannot possibly calculate perfectly every time. It is the continuous and sustained highs or lows that cause complications over time. Don't pressure yourself too much. Please understand that, despite the grim statistics and discouraging news we diabetics are bombarded with on an almost daily basis, diabetes is not a death sentence, and complications are not a given. In many ways, you can choose how healthy you are. If you have been recently diagnosed, take the necessary steps to educate

116

yourself and learn about your body now, and you won't have to fear complications later. If you have had diabetes for years, and perhaps even have a few complications, realize that many complications can potentially be reversed if you can gain good control of your diabetes. From climbing mountains to having babies, a healthy diabetic in good control can do almost anything a non-diabetic can; it simply requires a bit more preparation. Of course, you may always be faced with the potential of a severe low or high, but mortality is a fact of life. As diabetics, we can only do our very best. Personally, I choose to live a full, enjoyable life while I aim for tight control. It is much more rewarding than the alternatives. Do the best you can. Then, don't forget to enjoy life and live each day to its fullest!

Appendixes

The following are tips and lists included to help you with daily life. They may be copied by the purchaser of this book, for personal use only. They are based on personal experiences and the experiences of the doctors and fellow diabetics I have conversed with over the years. You should have the list approved by your doctor, modifying it as necessary for your personal needs.

Appendix A: *Low BG Treatments*

There are many options for treating a low blood sugar level, and you should discuss these options with your doctor. To give you some ideas, I have listed a few of my favorites here, as well as treatments often recommended by doctors and nutritionists. Remember to test your BG about 30 minutes after trying a new treatment in order to make adjustments to the amounts suggested here.

- ½ cup orange or apple juice
- ¼ cup grape juice
- 6 ounce Glucerna shake
- ½ banana, large apple, orange, pear, etc.
- ½ cup of grapes or strawberries
- ½ cup ice cream
- Hard candy (as specified by your doctor)
- Glucose tablets
- Glucose gel
- Small Fruit bar or 2 Fig newtons
- ½ standard sized candy bar or ¼ of a king-sized bar
- ½ cup regular soda

Appendix B: *"Safe" and Low-carb Munchies*

- Cheese Slice
- Cheese Sticks
- Jerky
- Carrots, celery, squash, radish, broccoli, etc. (with or without a non-sweet, vegetable dip)
- Celery (with or without Peanut Butter with no added sugar)
- Sugarless Gum
- Sugarless, carb-free candies

Appendix C: *Record Keeping*

Discuss proper record keeping with your doctor, as each doctor has a preference regarding the data you record.

1. Tips for good record keeping:
   - Unless otherwise recommended by your doctor, test a minimum of four times per day, but not more than every two hours. Most doctors like you to test your BG level around 2:00 a.m., before breakfast, two hours after breakfast, before lunch, two hours after lunch, before dinner, two hours after dinner, and/or bedtime.
   - Try to test at the same time every day, particularly when trying to figure out your body's patterns and insulin needs.
   - Middle of the night tests may only be needed once or twice a week when BG levels are stable. It may help to drink a large glass of water before bed. The urge to urinate will help wake you.
   - For maintenance purposes, testing two hours after a meal may be rotated based on different days. For example, on Monday, test after breakfast; on Tuesday, test after lunch; on Wednesday, test after dinner; then start over again. This will give you two tests after each meal every week.
   - When you record an unusual BG level, record the reason (if known) in the notes section under the BG level. For example,

you may mention "forgot to bolus," "washed the car," or "sat in an airplane for four hours." This will help your doctor decide which BG levels should be ignored and which levels require a change in your insulin levels.

- Record keeping can be a monotonous and boring task, so ask your doctor if it is acceptable to record everything one time each day-- such as before bed.

- If you have the software or capability to create your own graphs from your BG levels, I recommend doing so. Even if your doctor doesn't use the graph, it can be very informative for you. A graph that has a line through the average levels makes it easy to figure out which BG numbers should be discounted, and which should be considered for a change in insulin. There are times when you may feel your BG levels are on a roller-coaster, but the graph may show there is simply a slight increase or decrease at certain times every day.

The following page is a simple log sheet similar to what I have used for years, and most of the doctors I have had appreciated the simplicity of it. It can be easily duplicated and expanded by creating a text and data table on your computer.

Name: _____

Date Range: _____

Time	A.M.	Brkfst	Mid	Lunch	P.M.	Dinner	Bed
BG							
Insulin							
Notes							
BG							
Insulin							
Notes							
BG							
Insulin							
Notes							
BG							
Insulin							
Notes							
BG							
Insulin							
Notes							
BG							
Insulin							
Notes							
BG							
Insulin							
Notes							

Appendix D: *Medical Packing List and Travel Tips*

1. Packing List
   - Meds or insulin with an extra two day supply for every seven days you are expecting to be gone (always better to error on the side of caution) Note: it is recommended to find a way to keep insulin cool. The label should have a suggested temperature range to help you.
   - Pump supplies with an extra set for every three sets you pack
   - Syringes: the number should be based on the number you anticipate using, plus an additional one or two per week
   - Meter and test kit, with an extra bottle of test strips for each trip (you may need to buy yourself time to see a doctor for a new prescription, or even to get through a holiday weekend when pharmacies are closed).
   - Batteries for your meter and/or pump
   - Replacement lancets
   - Alcohol swabs/gauze
   - Log book
   - Medical ID bracelet or necklace, and appropriate medical ID and information cards should be worn or carried on your body
   - Customer service phone numbers for your meter, pump supplier, doctor, and pharmacy.
   - Glucagon injection (should be nearby at all times, with at least one person knowledgeable of how to use it)
   - Juice boxes

- Snacks (I prefer 6-packs of cheese or peanut crackers, due to their balance of protein and carbs, as well as their portability)
- Cash in the event of a low blood sugar or other emergency

2. Tips specific to air, train, or ship travel
    - Have your doctor write a note on professional stationary, with date and signature, certifying that you have diabetes. It should also include a brief description of your needed supplies. It is rare for anyone to request such an authorization, but always better safe than sorry. It is recommended to have this letter updated within 30 days of a trip, however, I experienced a case where it was usable within one year.
    - Diabetes is a disease protected by some of the laws of the Americans with Disabilities Act. As a result, you may be exempt from certain regulations. For example, when passing through a security checkpoint at an airport, if you are a Type 1 diabetic and regularly suffer from hypoglycemic reactions, you are allowed to carry juice boxes, and certain other sealed beverages, liquids, and gels, as long is you declare it and state your medical reason. A note from your doctor can help in these cases.
    - Also, thanks to the disability laws, if you are staying in a hotel, you may qualify for an in-room refrigerator at no charge in order to store your insulin. Ask the hotel service rep or manager for more information.

- Be sure to always include your medical supplies in carry-on luggage. You never want to risk losing it with any lost baggage. You can survive for a while without clothes or toiletries, but not without insulin!
- Learn your body's reaction to travel and be prepared to adjust accordingly.
- Talk with your doctor about international travel so you can be as prepared as possible for any delays or situations that may arise.

Appendix E: *Recommended Emergency Preparations*

1. Jewelry, medical ID, or other equipment to identify you as a diabetic. Some versions have a contact phone number where medical personnel can retrieve your medical information. I also recommend writing up an information card that is stored in your wallet or with your identification. In the event you are unable to communicate, this card should include your emergency contacts, your physician information, and a brief synopsis of your medical history. The medical history should include allergies, type of diabetes, year diagnosed, any complications, medications and insulin used, and daily insulin rates. If you use a pump, record the pre-set basal and bolus rates as well as the average daily rates. This will help the attending physician calculate your needed dosage in the event your pump is removed.

2. ICE (In Case of Emergency) contact name and number programmed into your cell phone.

3. A list of needed supplies stored in an accessible location for friends or family. I would list the number of supplies you would need for a one week period. While hospitals do stock supplies such as alcohol swabs, gauze, insulin, test strips, and syringes, it can require a great deal of "red tape" and lengthy wait times to get the items you need. Furthermore, the hospital may not stock the type of insulin, lancet, or test strip that you need. The list should include things such as the following:

- # of syringes
- # of pump reservoirs (if applicable)

- # of pump tubing sets (if applicable)
- # of insulin bottles and what kind
- # of bottles of test strips
- # of spare lancets
- Spare meter and test supplies (if applicable)
- # of spare batteries and what kind
- # of alcohol and gauze pads
- # of juice boxes or other portable low-sugar treatments
- The contact information for your regular doctor and diabetes specialists

4. Be sure to notify your chosen family or friends of the location of your list and all supplies so they can pack easily.

5. I included your test kit and low sugar treatments in this list because of personal experiences. Medical personnel are required to test your blood at certain intervals throughout the day. If you feel you are low or high, however, it can be difficult to get yourself tested because of hospital regulations. Additionally, if you are low and require treatment, it can sometimes be difficult to get help or the necessary supplies in a timely manner. As a general rule, the more self-sufficient you can be, the less stress you will experience. In fact, some hospitals will permit you to have (and may even supply) a mini-refrigerator in your hospital room to store juice and insulin. They may offer to store your supplies in the nurses' kitchen, but use caution. When I was hospitalized during my pregnancy, I had some insulin in the lounge

fridge thrown out by a cleaning crew. Self-sufficiency often shows medical personnel that you are very knowledgeable about your disease, and they will often be more cooperative and helpful as a result.

Appendix F: *Recommended Links for Additional Information*

- Insulin Pumps and Supplies: www.minimed.com
- Detailed Diabetes Information:
  www.diabetes-normalsugars.com
- The American Diabetes Association:
  www.diabetes.org
- Diabetes Basics:
  http://www.cdc.gov/diabetes/faq/basics.htm
- Nutritional Calculator:
  http://recipes.sparkpeople.com/recipe-calculator.asp

About the Author

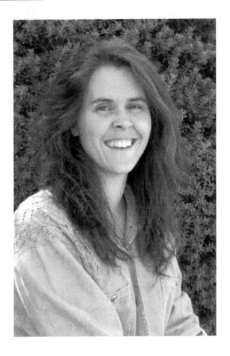

Danielle Londrigan was diagnosed with Type 1 diabetes in 1984. She was just four years old. Since that day, she has worked closely with her doctors to maintain tight control of her diabetes. Over the years, she has counseled with many professionals and other diabetics, in order to educate herself about the disease. Her efforts have certainly proven worthwhile.

Today, Danielle is an active wife and mother. Her husband, Sean, is active duty military, and they have four children. She stays busy homeschooling her children, educating others about diabetes, and free-lance writing.

Made in the USA
Columbia, SC
17 September 2022

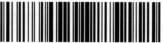

67416792R00076